MY
SECRETS OF
SURVIVORSHIP

MY

SECRETS OF
SURVIVORSHIP

WE SOLVED THE MYSTERY!

MELISSA MAE PALMER

MA in Professional Counseling

DAGOSTIN
PUBLISHING

My Secrets of Survivorship
Published by DAgostin Publishing

This book is designed to provide accurate and authoritative information with regard to the subject matter covered. This information is given with the understanding that neither the author nor publisher is engaged in rendering legal or professional advice. Since the details of your situation are fact dependent, you should additionally seek the services of a competent professional.

ISBN: 978-0-9986410-1-0

Printed in the United States of America

I would like to dedicate this book to my mother,
Nancy Grimes D'Agostin.
She taught me to love your family and believe in God.
If I can be half the mother you are, I will be complete.
This book is also dedicated to my five children
and my friends.

CONTENTS

FOREWORD

by Lynda Yost

I could never have imagined that I would learn so much from a young woman a generation younger than myself, a mother of five while I had none, a former career woman who gave it all up, and a person with more disposable income than myself. But I have.

The tie that binds Melissa Mae Palmer and Lynda Yost is also what allows us to manage stress—the love of fashion as a wearable art form and mode of self-expression. We have very different tastes in our fashion choices, but both of us use it as an escape for our adult issues, our career and parenting stress, and our time demands.

I first met Melissa four years ago when she and her husband moved in across the street from me and my husband. At that time they had an infant, Charlie, one child from Shawn's previous marriage, and one child from Melissa's previous marriage. This combined family is pretty normal, and I was pleased to see how the combined family was working. I witnessed a genuine love for each other's children as well as a protectiveness for their infant son. I was also managing a combined family after being single for twenty-five years. But things weren't quite as they seemed across the street from me.

When I had several neighbors over to introduce them to the Palmers, only Shawn showed up. Melissa had to stay home as she was pregnant and not up to a social function. During a similar social neighborhood dinner at my home several years later, Melissa announced that she was again pregnant, so she and Shawn would take turns coming over to the dinner party as one had to stay home to care for the other four children. Totally understandable, I thought, until I began to see Melissa out on the street side of her home watching for the school bus and walking very wobbly back to her house after the children were safely on the school bus. When I asked her about her gait, she said that she thought she had Lyme disease.

As our time together increased as we ran into each other getting the mail, Melissa confided more to me and opened up about her previous life as a medical device sales person and her tremendous financial success as such. I learned that she was a single parent for a very long time. I found out that she actually valued me as a friend despite our age difference and lifestyles. I knew I had to start helping Melissa deal with her health issues when her daughter asked me if I was ever going to move. It seems that her daughter knew my home had a first-floor bedroom, and her mother was no longer able to climb the stairs to the master bedroom in her home. If they could move across the street to my home, the other children could stay in the school district, and Melissa wouldn't have to climb stairs. This conversation was a wake-up call for me. This wasn't Lyme disease; it was something much more unusual and serious.

So I invited Melissa over to see my closet showroom and tell her about my past career as a pioneering woman executive that became the head of a Fortune 500 company at the young age of thirty-seven. I told her that since I had no children, I was enjoying watching her family grow. As I showed her my vintage couture collection of clothing, I let her know that I was now retired, no longer watching out the window of a home office, and instead was following my passion for fashion. She said that she admired my intelligence and flamboyant fashion tastes and wanted me to help her with fashion and family advice. I was so flattered that I decided we would be friends forever, and I would be her confidant.

Little did I know that as Melissa confided in me about her final diagnosis of Pompe disease I would be taking a journey of my own. I witnessed and learned from Melissa about the continuing need to be frank and forthcoming in one's relationships in order to have the support one needs for life's challenges. I saw that there are second chances in life if one can clearly define one's life goals just as she and I had defined career and business goals in our previous positions. I learned that girlfriends can compensate and provide understanding for the female point of view when our husbands just want to "fix" us. I learned to search for medical answers myself and to find alternative doctors' opinions when symptoms get worse and the treatment isn't working. And, finally, I have learned to accept what I cannot change and to move on.

I can read my Italian Vogue and Donna magazines, recall when I wore those types of clothes in my social and business life, but know that Melissa and I have both moved on. We cannot change the challenges we have both faced in our lives, but we know that our friends and the support systems we have built will work now and in the future.

If we need time to process our next move, we can just pick up a fashion magazine or take a walk in our closets to play with clothes and take a break from the reality of the choice we are pondering. We can call each other up and talk about the next event we will be going to and what we will wear. And then the next step in our life journey will come to us once that creative need for fashion has given us the calm we need to implement it.

Note:
Lynda Yost is the past president of World Dryer Corporation, the world leader in the manufacture of warm air hand dryers for public bathrooms. She is also the past president of the commercial divisions of The Thermos Company and Stanley Company. She has had her couture fashions from the 1980s and 1990s purchased by five museums and many Hollywood stars for red-carpet appearances. She continues to live across the street from Mellissa's previous home but maintains her constant communication with her young "friend for life."

- 1 -

Meet a Simple Girl

*Hiding secrets and white lies only causes anxiety
and low self-esteem.*

—*Melissa Mae Palmer*

My name is Melissa Mae Palmer. I was born September 20, 1973, to Edward and Nancy D'Agostin. My father, who lovingly calls me "Lissy," is a man's man who people can talk to for hours because his conversation is always engaging. He is a blast to be around, and Ed D'Agostin remembers everything about a person, which is what I believe made him so successful in his sales career. He remembers their names, children's names, and their favorite things to do. He sold capital printing equipment and was the top sales representative for three decades, and his career success, combined with my mother's nursing career, provided my siblings and me a stable, loving home. I was raised in a middle-class family in Hinckley, Ohio, and then Illinois, and my parents were always so loving. They are still together today, in fact. Just being around them has always made me happy; it still does. They have a dream marriage that is so wonderful to witness. The romance they exude makes me smile to this day after watching their love grow for forty-plus years. They still love each other like it was their wedding day. They also love all their children with all their hearts, just as they did the day we were all born. That love has inspired a lot in my life.

I'm the oldest of three, and I suppose that is why I may at times seem a little bossy. I have a brother, Billy, who is three years my junior, and a sister, Mary, who is five years younger than me. Billy is a giant man just like my father. He looks like him in almost every way, but my brother has some special needs. Mary, on the other hand, looks like my paternal grandmother. They both still live at home with my parents, who are now in Florida after having lived in Illinois for years. They are waiting for that special man and woman to come along so they can strive to create what our parents have—a beautiful marriage with a beautiful family. I am the only one who has given my parents grandchildren so far, but I have given them five beautiful grandchildren to carry on their legacy, which is priceless.

My family lived in Hinckley, Ohio, for years when I was a child. It was in Ohio I learned to conceal my mystery symptoms. As far back as I can remember, I knew that I had a problem with my health, but for reasons I still cannot explain, I hid them from other people, even physicians. I would not recommend to anyone to do this, but I did. I lied to doctors and my parents for as early as I could remember, and my mother is a nurse. I was in and out of the hospital a couple of times after my eighth birthday. I knew that there was something different about me—something that was perplexing even to medical professionals. First of all, I had diarrhea every single morning of my life. I was also always exhausted, and I had pain all over. My defense was to combat these symptoms for reasons that I will explain, but I promise there is an answer in my voyage. I felt bad,

I did not know what do with my pleaser personality, and I never complained to anyone. No matter how many times I went and how many tests were run, I always left the doctors scratching their heads, more or less, and I never seemed to get any better. I was a mystery to everyone and even myself. I have struggled with pain and fatigue for as long as I can remember, but I never told anyone about it, ever. I questioned if it was real, and I was not honest with anyone about the pain and suffering I was going through from the time I was in grade school. It was difficult to be a little girl and feel sick and hide it from everyone. I had anxiety and low self-esteem as a child because I never felt good, and I kept it to myself. I'm a fighter, and I have been since I was just a smiling little girl with dark-brown eyes and chocolate-colored hair. I was always extremely petite, but my little secret kept me tinier than most. I did all I could to keep anyone from knowing why I was so tiny.

It got tougher to hide as time went by. I did everything to hide these profound symptoms by sleeping on desktops and not eating, but there was no way to conceal them entirely. I was diagnosed with scoliosis, and once my fifth-grade teacher named Mr. Cirt in Hinckley, Ohio, asked me why I used the powder room so much. I was good at thinking on my toes, and I made up an excuse so I could continue to keep this a secret from my hippie parents to continue to protect them. That was right before we moved to Illinois, to the posh suburb Barrington, in middle school, which was close to culture shock. I was not aware that designer clothes existed, but I learned quickly. I had to say good-bye to my childhood best friend named Niki and leave her heartbroken at twelve years old. I did not like it one bit at first, and the only time that I visited the school nurse in this posh upscale suburb was to have my mother leave work as a nurse and pick me up from school because I missed Niki and I did not fit in. I cried my eyes out every day. I wanted to move back to Hinckley, Ohio. Middle school in Barrington, Illinois, was not the perfect time to move, but with the right group of friends, I made the best out of it. I was accepted by a wonderful, little crowd, which made it much easier to be middle class in an upscale area.

We moved into our house, and I met these girls; their names were Heidi, Nola, Emily, and Deanna. We named our group the BOD squad. We all lived about twenty minutes in far north in Barrington where all of our classmates spent time together on the weekends, but we were far enough away from one another that we could not walk or ride our bikes to each other. That meant that we would do sleepovers every weekend we were together. During the week at school, we were also inseparable. We had a bond like sisters, if not stronger. We all knew who everyone else liked and did not like, and we stuck up for each other without hesitation. We were like a family; nothing got between us.

The times I spent with BOD were some of the best times of my adolescence. We would do silly things that all teenagers do. In middle school, we would prank call all the pizza joints and Chinese restaurants around town. We took turns talking in funny voices to the person unlucky enough to answer the phone. When we were younger, we had some friends that were boys, but they were the film crowd, and once they had girlfriends, they did not spend time with us anymore. We didn't care though; we had each other, and we had plenty of fun without them—sometimes too much fun. Once when I was house-sitting we all got drunk, and Nola humped a ceramic frog. Needless to say, the frog did not make it thought the episode. I was stuck with a broken frog with no explanation. I knew I was going to be in big trouble, but I admitted what I had done the second the homeowners returned. I've always been quick to admit when I am wrong. I couldn't stand lying. I would come clean about everything at the drop of a hat.

"I'm so sorry," I told Mrs. Jones, the homeowner. She was the mother of one of Billy's friends. "I had a little gathering with my friends, and we ended up drinking your alcohol and making a lot of phone calls. I will pay for everything, I promise."

We ended up with a one-hundred-dollar phone bill, which I paid just as I promised. She could see how awful I felt for not being responsible when she trusted me, so she told me that she would not tell my parents. And she kept that promise. To this day I try to pay it forward through parenting from the lesson that I had learned from her. I always learn the hard way with life. My father says that I learned every lesson, and I do. I am honest, and I always stand up and apologize.

So although I did get in a little bit of trouble here and there with my squad, they were ultimately one of the best things that ever happened to me. We watched Heathers, 90210, Sixteen

16

Candles, and the Breakfast Club a hundred times together, and we had a rule that we were never ever to date another member's man. I knew I always had someone on my side because of them and that I could tell them anything. Still, however, I kept one big secret from them. I kept that huge secret that there was always something that made life hard for me—the secret I kept for thirty-six years until I collapsed in the arms of a beloved doctor, Dr. McDonough, who is a true angel in my life. I will explain why in depth later.

I had symptoms of a mysterious illness for so many years, but I never said a thing to anyone about it, not even the BOD squad. I even lied to protect my family. My parents are so wonderful, and had they known about my severe health issues they would have taken me to the doctor immediately, but I did everything I could to keep it from them. I had diarrhea every time I ate, scoliosis, pain, weakness, and raging liver enzymes, but I made it my life's goal to keep all of it to myself. I told my mother the scoliosis test must've been wrong, and I used every excuse possible to hide the symptoms.

I fought to live a normal life and did everything I could to survive without burdening anyone around me. We already had a family situation with Billy that kept us busy. He has learning disabilities, but my parents were hippies and did not believe in getting him treatment. Instead, they believed in natural remedies, which is bizarre because my mom was a surgical nurse with a scientific edge. They tried to be as natural as possible, however. We would drive him an hour to a school that was different from other schools. Having a child with some special needs makes it difficult for a family. We were different from others in Cleveland, Ohio. My dad would take forty vitamins a day and make raw juices. Vitamins and carrot juice never really helped Billy's behavioral problems, however. He has spent his life making poor decisions that I or my parents would have to bail him out of. I opted to stay silent about my symptoms because of that, among other things. I coped with, ignored, and hid the pain and fatigue I dealt with daily and worked hard to achieve the dream of getting married to a wonderful man and having amazing children. I just wanted to attain the American

Dream, and I wasn't going to let whatever was causing all my problems stop me.

What is interesting about my own mystery illness—and my mother's aversion to modern medicine—is that my maternal grandmother, Catherine, lived a lot of her life with severe muscular pain that went undiagnosed. She was in a wheelchair from the time she was only fifty years old. When I was a little girl, my grandma explained to me on more than one occasion that good girls are seen and not heard, and her words were the gospel to me. I loved and admired her so much that I eventually named my youngest daughter after her. That little adage made its mark on me, and so I suffered in silence, just as my grandma did.

My maternal grandfather, who was fifteen years older than my grandmother, died when I was only three months old of a heart attack, so I never knew him, although I have heard countless stories about how wonderful he was and how much everyone loved him. He and my grandmother came from Czechoslovakia. He was educated and trained as a teacher but worked for Chevrolet in LaGrange, Illinois, for the benefits. When he retired, he spent as much time as he could with my grandmother and mother; he would hold my mother on his lap as my grandmother cooked amazing gourmet meals. My grandma was so depressed when she lost my grandfather, who was truly the love of her life. Between the depression and the chronic pain, she had to live with my mother's oldest sister, my Aunt Kathy, because she could no longer take care of herself. Shortly after her father's death, my mother, who is the youngest of her three siblings, had to move to Ohio for my father's first job. I was three months old at the time. My grandmother stayed with my Aunt Kathy for the rest of her life, which she lived out in pain that no doctor could ever diagnose. Each physician assumed it was seronegative arthritis when they could not figure anything else out. I never considered that perhaps the same pain that plagued me was related to my grandmother's pain. All I knew as a child was that my grandmother was always in a rocking chair or a wheelchair when we would visit her and that I loved her very much. She probably had my illness; she had all the symptoms, and it is all in our genetics. We are what our genetics say we are.

Like my grandmother, I spent my life in pain, but I made sure no one knew. Things that were easy for others were grueling for me, so I fought just to keep up with everyone else while achieving all my goals and desires. I learned well how to pretend to feel good when I did not. There was always a good reason that I did not feel good. My health was always in peril because I had a major disease. I knew that to some degree, although I was not sure at all what disease it was. I just concealed it for survival. I learned to live with discomfort for the sake of others. I learned to be a survivor for my family; first it was my parents, then my own husband and children. I lied about follow-up doctors' visits, and I fought all the ailments—all the pain and fatigue that made getting out of bed a chore as difficult as running five miles—and then I collapsed at Dr. McDonough's office. This was after my last childbirth. This is my story, about how I got to where I am today. It is a story of survival—not once, but two times over. Just like a cat, I have nine lives, but my nine lives have come from divine intervention. Once you see my weird science, you will agree. It is also the story of a rare genetic code that has perplexed doctors to date. You see, even after I was finally diagnosed and we figured out the mystery illness after decades of not knowing and searched for a cure when I would graduate college at Northern Illinois University and get health insurance (I knew then I would find the answer), I continued to be an enigma. Read on and you will find out why.

Tips for Survivorship, Part 1

1. Do not suffer in silence.

Pain, weakness, and diarrhea caused me to have low self-esteem and anxiety as a child. Do not hide your illness. I was a little girl that could not carry laundry upstairs. I was always tired and could not eat. I did not tell anyone because of my brother, Billy. Put yourself first.

2. Friends make everything better.

I had my best friend Niki in Ohio until sixth grade. I also found my group in high school. Illness is better with fun times. Watch Breakfast Club, Heathers, and tease boys; laughter takes away stress.

3. Find a confidant who inspires you.

Grandma Catherine was an inspiration to me. I would confide in her about her illness. We all need someone to relate with. She never knew how horrible I felt, and if she did, she would have cared because I was very close with her. I knew that I had the same illness that she had.

4. Pray constantly.

My family are all Christians; prayer every night helped me achieve my goals in life.

5. Look for role models.

Admiring my father, Edward D'Agostin Jr., and cleaning our house every Saturday gave me a foundation for hard work and setting goals. He was my role model.

- 2 -

Surviving and Thriving

Life was in the way of a cure for me. Goals, babies, and my career took the forefront. I was not ready to fall in love, but I fell in love with my "rock." We can never control our passion, desire, and love.

—*Melissa Mae Palmer*

At age thirty, I was a single mother with a beautiful eight-year-old daughter named Taylor Mae from a previous marriage. God blessed me with the news of her two months after I graduated from college. It wasn't a planned pregnancy by any means. I got pregnant by a man named Mark, the high school football star who never talked to me when we were in school together. These were the parties that the BOD squad and I never attended, but we sure wanted to. I guess you would call them the popular crowd parties, and the BOD squad never attended them.

I had a fabulous dream after college to get a job with health insurance and find out my mysterious symptoms, and then I found out I was having a baby unexpectedly. Her name is Taylor Mae, and she was a surprise, but the best surprise of my life. Together, we told my father the news after the Atlanta Braves won the World Series. My dad was in a state of bliss that I had graduated from his college and had a lucrative sales job in Chicago with Authorized Medical Scope Repair. Mark strategically told him the news that a little baby was coming in nine months just after he watched his Atlanta Braves win the World Series. My dad has a passion for baseball, so he was in a wonderful mood, then he found out his oldest daughter was pregnant. He looked back at us with an expression of disappointment, but he welcomed Taylor.

I married Mark, and we had Taylor. After she was five weeks old, we moved to Arizona. Mark had a business deal with my father that fell through. I was the one making the money in our home, so I had to keep my job. I was the top sales representative at Medical Scope Repair and doing very well financially. Mark made the poverty line, but he was able to carry health insurance for us while we were married. I was number one in sales every month. The apple does not fall far the tree; just like my father, I achieved in my sales job, but Mark wanted to achieve as well. The TV was his favorite thing to do, however, except when Taylor came into this world. He was in love with her and told her that she would go to his college, the University of Iowa, and eventually she did even, though she spent little time with him throughout her childhood.

He wanted to try to succeed in Arizona, and I agreed that when Taylor was old enough, we would move. After each pregnancy I would crash with this super mysterious illness. I had a really mystery brewing with my health—or was it in my head?

At six months pregnant, I found out from my father-in-law, who was a business owner, that my company could not legally fire me for being pregnant. I told my manager, who said she would make sure I was protected. I explained to her that I had been the top sales rep and was excelling at my job and that I had no intentions of slowing down. I had a great reputation with doctors and nurses all around the region. I was also getting calls from medical recruiters around Chicago.

"I will need four weeks off for maternity leave, but after that I will be back and working just as hard as ever," I assured her.

My manager said she would take care of me, but once I told her they split my territory up and hired another sales representative. I was proud of all I had accomplished, but I felt like I was always on the verge of being pushed out.

As we awaited the arrival of my little blessing from above, my dad suggested that Mark start go into business with him opening up a Packmail so he could finally support our family, especially since I would be on maternity leave for a month. He agreed it was a good idea and was excited, but they lost the lease to Barnes and Noble, and so the entire deal fell through. Mark was back at square one, and I was still breadwinner, as always. All the symptoms I had suffered since I was a girl were gone, so I had more energy than usual. I worked around the clock up until the moment my water broke while I was standing in a Nordstrom with my boss, who was disgusted at the fluid that came gushing out of me at Woodfield Mall in Schaumburg, Illinois. My boss could afford Nordstrom, but I was having the most beautiful gift from God that was better than money; it was priceless. Even though I was twenty-two years old, I was ready for Taylor, and I knew that I could handle her even if Mark and I didn't work out. I grew up babysitting. I'm the oldest of three, and I love children. I had the best family as well, which set a great example.

I had my daughter young—at twenty-two years old. When most women my age were out barhopping, I was preparing for my firstborn. I was scared, but the moment I saw the porcelain-skinned, blonde-haired little girl that I had worked for twenty-two grueling hours to give birth to, I knew that I had found a new reason to be my best. Taylor made me fight to thrive, and I did. I sent myself to graduate school. After that, I managed not only to make it in corporate America as a single mother parenting alone, but to become a self-made millionaire. What is so significant about my success, however, isn't that I was able to do it as a young, single mother. Sure, that part added obstacles that few of my peers faced, but that was hardly the toughest part of my battle. My daughter was an inspiration for me to do better; my health, however, was a constant war. I say *war* instead of battle for good reason.

The reprieve I had enjoyed while pregnant vanished after I had Taylor Mae. In fact, the symptoms came back with a vengeance. I had signs of illness early in life, but I always hid them. I told only one person from the time I was a child until I was finally forced to share my secret, and his name was Jerry, but that wasn't until I was in college at Arizona State, and it went no further than the two of us. I have mentioned this to three top genetic physicians, and there has been no response. Why, during pregnancy, would I have no symptoms for this profound illness?

"Why not tell your parents?" Jerry asked when I told him. He had met them, and he knew how terrific they were. My mom was always concerned about how thin I was and always asked if I was eating. I assured her I was, but the truth was I couldn't because food would upset my stomach, and I would feed my dogs under the table.

"I know that they would understand," I replied. "But they have Billy to deal with. He's always causing so much trouble, and I cannot disappoint them."

"But you have to tell them about this," he insisted.

"I'm tough, and I can handle it," I retorted. My defense mechanism was to put everything that was negative at the back of my mind. I certainly wasn't going to tell others about it.

It is important to have friends when you have a secret. Jerry was a secret to my survivorship because I could talk to him about my perceived illness, and he was the only friend ever. His mother had passed away from cancer when he was six years old, so he was extremely understanding of illness. I leaned on him and no one else, hoping that I'd figure out some day what was wrong with me. Here are the accommodations that he made for our platonic friendship. He bought comfortable pillows for his bed; big, soft blankets; and wonderful sheets. Now we were *broke* college kids. We remained friends for most of our lifetime.

After I told Jerry about it, he would always ask me if I was okay when we would eat. We had the best friendship in the world. He always looked out for my symptoms of pain, weakness, and my upset stomach. I would sleep alone in his comfortable bed with memory foam pillows and a feather blanket that helped with the spinal pain I had. It seemed to make my symptoms easier to deal with when I had someone to share my secret with. All those years of being alone with the secret of my illness made me scared and lonely, but finally I had a very special friendship. The security and honesty we shared was something that I'll never forget. It was really great to have a friend to share my big secret with, and he never told a soul. Neither did I. A best friend can see the truth and pain of illness when you are fooling the world. That was Jerry. He knew my embarrassing secrets and made accommodations for me—that is what a best friend can do when you are surviving an illness. You don't have to do it alone, and you shouldn't.

While I was at college at Arizona, I realized that the sun was healing for me. When I would lie out, I felt less symptomatic. It was probably the vitamin D deficiency that I have. Then one day I met someone with chronic fatigue syndrome at the pool at Arizona State University. I started talking to this pretty girl that was at one of the dorm pools, and she told me she had chronic fatigue syndrome. I asked her what her symptoms were. The fatigue part was so much like mine. She was always tired, and so was I. She would take one class and sleep for hours. I could not do that, however, so I started drinking coffee around the clock to stay awake. I was only at Arizona a year, however, and then I was back home after wasting my parents' money on tuition because I knew everything about Long Island and I had a lot of fun. I got a job and went to the community college called Harper, and I continued to keep my secret, not without Jerry to talk to. I had too much fun at Arizona State to voyage back to Chicago and pay my own way through college because of the sunbathing and lack of studying. My parents were disappointed. I figured out that waitressing was the most effective way to earn money and work less. My parents made me—and deservingly so—cover my expenses as a result of screwing up my freshman year in college. I accepted the result of my actions and worked hard because I knew that I screwed up, and hard work is one thing that I know how to do best. In life, I learned every lesson the hard way. I enjoyed meeting professionals at my three waitressing jobs. They inspired me, as my father did, to someday make it in corporate America.

I ended up waitressing throughout my college days. I made it to Northern Illinois University, where I eventually graduated with a degree in psychology. This made both my parents very proud, but my job, on the other hand, did not. I ended up taking a job at Hooters to help pay for college, and I kept it from my parents the entire time. They were ultraconservative, and I knew they wouldn't approve. Then my W2 came and let my secret out. They were as angry as I thought they'd be, but in my defense I was keeping up with my studies, keeping a job, and driving to and from Dekalb, Illinois, which was an hour from Barrington. Yes, I was a Hooters girl, but orange shorts through college and spending money is all that it meant for me, right? *Wrong.* Unfortunately, it meant so much more to my parents. Again I disappointed them.

Still, I was a girl with a purpose, and that was to figure out my illness. I made it through my last year drinking coffee constantly, getting as much sun as I could to ease my symptoms, and sleeping in my car between classes, but I made it! I was determined to fight for what I wanted, and I did what I set out to do.

I knew that it was time to get health insurance and work to find out what was wrong with me and search for a diagnosis because I knew there was something different about me, and it was not caused by those teenage years of puberty and hormones. I needed to find out why I felt so bad all the time; coffee and sun were not going to cut it anymore. I remembered my liver enzymes being high and always having scoliosis as a child. My goal was to find out where these mysterious symptoms were coming from, and health insurance was going to be the answer. I was inspired to get health insurance because I never felt good. It is called *malaise.* You feel like something is totally wrong. I was ready to find out what it was, but then my parents sent me to Las Vegas as a graduation gift. My mother bought me a perfect navy suit to interview in and a briefcase. It was the best gift ever because I knew that I needed to find a career, but it also put my health on the backburner once again.

My mother, Nancy, has been the best person in my life. Behind every female is a strong mother. Mine showed me how to love and trust. I'm very lucky to have her, and I love her more than anything. She taught me to be honest and polite. To love others and money is not important. What is important are your inner feelings of security, and you get that from love.

I took a position at Authorized Scope Repair, which was one hundred percent commission and no health insurance. I was so proud of myself, and in three months I was making a lot of money with this one-hundred-percent commission job. I saved the hospitals thousands of dollars by gathering scopes with high-tech video equipment in them to be repaired instead of sending them back to the manufacturer. I was never so excited in my life about a job. It was a new innovative idea. My boss was this beautiful female who moved to Chicago to be close to me. We became best friends. Everything was going great, but it was a new company and they did not offer health insurance, so I was still dodging my illness. I continued to survive in every way I could until I could finally get into someone to help get me some answers.

I thought that after college graduation I would have health insurance and that I would find out the answers that I needed, but life kept getting in the way. In a strange way, I am thankful for that. My father always said that everything in my life I learn the hard way. I learned to survive, and I was able to see everything I was capable of, but the fact remained: I was sick and didn't know why. Why could I not climb the stairs without holding on to the railing? I could never blow up a balloon. When I was tired, people would ask, "Why are you limping?" These symptoms were profound, and, yes, I was exhausted. I wanted to go to bed by 8:00 p.m. every night. Why? There had to be a reason.

When I had a child at a young age who depended solely on me, it became even more important to me to hide any weakness because I did not want to go home and live with my parents. I knew from childhood that I had an illness, but I did not want to know what. Feeling bad all of time gave me a great deal of anxiety. That perceived weakness became my little secret, and I had no intentions of sharing it with anyone until I was fully ready to do so. The problem was, I never seemed to feel ready to tell others about my chronic pain, weakness, and severe diarrhea. How could I not have low self-esteem? I could not go on a date and eat for the fright of having diarrhea. It was awful to live like this.

Mark and I had moved to Arizona together shortly after we had Taylor Mae. I had gotten a job almost immediately with McKesson HBOC, so I was making decent money, but Mark was having trouble finding a job. He decided to work odd jobs that didn't make much money when he did get them, and I worked as hard as I could to keep us afloat and take care of Taylor. My symptoms were in full swing by that time, so everything became so much harder to handle. Every pregnancy I felt great, and then I would crash with my symptoms after I gave birth. Were the babies giving me an unidentified enzyme?

I did much of the caring for Taylor as I worked around the clock. I thank God to this day that she was such a wonderful baby that enjoyed her sleep. Taylor still sleeps more than anyone I know. Even though Taylor did sleep well, she still needed me for everything, and I was fighting exhaustion and chronic pain every minute of the day. I finally went to a general physician in Arizona about six weeks after having Taylor for help only to have him diagnose me with depression. He claimed it was related to giving birth and put me on Prozac. He said I'd feel fine in six weeks. I began to question my sanity at that point. I had finally told a doctor of some of my symptoms, only to be told it was in my head. The diagnosis was postpartum depression. I was getting ready to get back to work seven weeks after having Taylor. Our family needed health insurance and money. It was sad; there we were in Arizona with no family. I had an aunt living there, but she was the superintendent of Maricopa County. She worked around the clock.

As I waited for the Prozac to make all my symptoms fade away, Mark and I got divorced. It happened after I overheard him describing his fun times at a bachelor party. Mark did indeed tell on himself. I wrapped Taylor Mae in a blanket, packed our things, and we began a new life together. I was a single mother without any family nearby. I walked down the street in the middle of the night and called a cab. I voyaged back to Chicago, where I called my boss. He said to take as much time off as possible and that my job was waiting for me in Phoenix. Wow, there are fabulous people in this universe.

Being a single mother left me with a lot of pressure to succeed, but I had my father's natural sales ability, and I learned to compensate. I worked smart. I could sleep two hours in the afternoon after work and before I picked up Taylor from daycare. But still, I was left in Arizona alone, dealing with an illness that I had no clue how to control and raising a child by myself. Being a single mother is no easy task anyway. It was particularly difficult for me since I was so far from my support system. I faced a lot of challenges because I did not live by any family to help me out with Taylor. There I was with no family in Arizona and all the responsibility of a child with a profound mysterious illness; this all kept me fighting for survival until one day, when I met Dr. Hoban. I decided to visit a physician again, a gastroenterologist. I worked in Chicago selling the service of repairing colonoscopies. I thought if diarrhea was a symptom, why not go to a gastroenterologist?

Dr. Hoban was amazing. The first thing he did was draw my blood and take a health history. He thought it was ulcerative colitis because a family member had it and my liver enzymes were raging. The labs came back and he said, "Your liver is sure angry with something."

He was the first one I was honest about my illness because he was nice and he believed in me. He called me and he said, "You have a problem."

"What is the problem?" I asked.

"Your liver enzymes are too high, and we need to get to the bottom of this," he told me. "Let's schedule a colonoscopy."

I was leery. After working with scope repair service in Chicago, I said to myself that I would never have one. I trusted Dr. Hoban, however, so I did.

Mark took me, and everything came back normal, but I had the elevated liver enzymes and the symptoms of diarrhea, pain, and weakness. Next, Dr. Hoban asked me to get my gallbladder checked out. It was working at thirteen percent, so I had to meet with a general surgeon. Dr. Hoban was sincerely concerned about me. He asked the general surgeon to perform a liver biopsy when he was taking out my gallbladder. The results came back, and my liver was *normal* despite the elevated liver enzymes. Dr. Hoban and I did not understand this.

Life got in the way again. I received a call from a recruiter in Phoenix; it was a sales representative with IV catheters. I was blessed with my career, and I owe it all to Taylor. I worked hard, and I was concerned about her. Before I was hired, I needed a physical. My liver enzymes came back high, and I was informed of the results. I had to stop searching for a cure to take care of Taylor. I needed this job and thought that this was my way to get transferred back to my family in Chicago. I sat down with Dr. Hoban to tell him my plans. I winked and said, "I have to raise my daughter. This is not the time to dig deeper. Let's just leave it alone."

I would see Dr. Hoban when I was in the hospital in Phoenix. I perplexed him with my unexplained lab results. He asked me how I was feeling, and I said, with a wink, that some things are better left alone.

I had to provide for my family. My life was good with Johnson and Jonson. With a traveling sales position, you do have a lot of freedom with your time. I would work smart and bypass a lunch. I could squeeze in a nap before I picked up Taylor. The schedule worked for me, although I had no girlfriends because of the demands of being a single mother and work. After work, I dedicated two hundred percent of my time to Taylor. I still was sick, but the good was better than the lifetime of undiagnosed symptoms.

I decided to go and pay cash to see a natural physician about my symptoms. My parents were thrilled that I went to an organic physician at a naturopathic clinic for my health issues and undiagnosed illness. It was there that I met a physician who was the director of the naturopathic college and also a trained osteopathic doctor. For the sake of the story, I refer to him as Dr. Organic.

He asked me to dinner after an appointment, and I agreed. One dinner led to another, and another. I loved spending time with him, and he loved spending time with me. We were both getting to know one another. We had some truly amazing times discussing politics, making dinner, talking about all our dreams and fears, and developing into a couple. There were some problems that surfaced, however, that I eventually had to face. For one, he was much older than I was—eighteen years older to be exact. I was fine with the age difference, but what I could not get over was that he never wanted anything to do with Taylor; he just wanted me. I would see him during the times Taylor was with her father, which was twice a week. This was the first man that I was alone with, and I enjoyed it, but I had little time to spend with him. As a single mother, you do the best that you can with the time that you have.

During my time in Arizona, Billy came to stay with me; he was helpful because I traveled with my sales career to Las Vegas. The Chicago sales manager at Johnson and Johnson was promoted to manager. I was the only single mom on the sales force. It was time to go back to Chicago and to be with my family. I was transferred home right before Taylor started kindergarten, and I was blessed. I mentioned to Dr. Organic I was moving in four days.

"What?" he said, and his face turned ghost white. It was the end of our relationship. I accepted that this man did not want to marry me because I was a single mom, and he did not want my most important fruit.

"Dr. Organic, you may want to be alone, but I do not," I told him. "Somewhere, someone is going to accept Taylor, and we are finished."

As a single mother, I should never have dated a man who did not want my entire package, but I did. I felt as a single mother that was what I was worth, but I was worth so much more. Just like that, I left him to be with my family who I had spent five years away from.

- 3 -

Making a New Life

The man that hit my car said to me, "I'm really sorry," and it was easy to accept his sincere apology. I could see the sincerity in his eyes. Everyone makes mistakes in life, and an apology is all that is needed.

—Melissa Mae Palmer

Six months after my move back to Chicago, I was blindsided by a terrible car accident that would lead to even more health issues.

To add to an already tough situation with graduate school and learning my new job with Johnson and Johnson in Chicago, I was hit head on by a Bobcat at fast food restaurant in Chicago after I picked up my sister Mary from my parents' house. I ended up having three shoulder surgeries, that last of which ended in a staph infection. I developed a pain condition called Complex Regional Pain Syndrome (CRPS), and I met my champion, who is Dr. Tim Lubenow, Director of Pain at Rush University.

The driver of the Bobcat settled out of court because it was clear I had sustained a lifelong injury. The settlement was hardly worth the scars and the constant, burning pain in my right shoulder, but I survived it all, and the settlement allowed me to pay off my school loans for graduate school from Illinois School of Professional Psychology and buy a house in Barrington, Illinois, where I was raised and where my father could stop by unexpected and brighten my day. I was excited about the tiny house that was perfect for us. Also, I was excited about graduate school and becoming a therapist. I love to help others, and I did my practicum with the physically and sexually abused.

"We are going to buy Taylor and you a house, pay off your school loans, and you are going to pretend that you do not have your settlement," my father said to me when we found out about the settlement. "You will put the rest of the money back in case you need it for medical care in the future. You can live off the interest."

He didn't want me to blow the money at Nordstrom buying gifts for other people or on charities. My father is a strong figure in my life, and I basically listen to every word that he says to me. He also knew that he was the only person I would listen to.

Okay," I agreed. "That's what I'll do."

It was a large Cook County settlement for the injury, which took me from rags to riches.

"Lissy, you are not giving anyone a penny," he admonished. "I love you, Lissy, but you make horrible choices with friends and men, and over my dead body will I see you give the money away."

I had never had any money in my entire life, so having a large sum at one time was new to me because I was always broke. I was more than happy to have my father's advice and his help. He set up a meeting with a financial firm in the Chicago. The check went straight to them. First, they paid my medical bills and then my attorney. I was recovering to some degree, and so I thought, *Nah, this isn't the time.*

I had just gotten out of a relationship with a man who turned out not to be quite who I thought he was. I found drugs in his pockets one day and knew it was time to end it. It was a real blow to me because before him I had been in a relationship with a man I truly loved and wanted to marry but who obviously did not have the same vision. None of that mattered now, however. We finally had our own home together, Taylor and me. It was a small, simple, ranch-style house, but perfectly ours. Every room was pink, and I added a hot tub and patio to sit and read in the summer as Taylor danced and did gymnastics in the backyard. But as perfect as everything was, all my milestones were sullied by my little secret—the nagging pain and relentless tiredness that put me in bed by eight every night with my daughter.

I was still struggling in graduate school at Illinois School of Professional Psychology, especially as I was forced to take out student loans from private banks, but I always finish a commitment.

Mystery of My Health

Year after year, as my health remained stable and my pain only got more intense, I told myself that I would expose my secret when the right time presented itself. The "right time" to me meant that all my family was ready to hear it. I could always find some reason not to tell, however. Either times were good and I didn't want to create waves or there was a family hardship—another illness, financial trouble, or maybe a death—and I didn't want to add to the chaos. At the end of the day, I felt ashamed of my illness, and I didn't want to share it with anyone. I didn't want people to look at me differently or to see me as anything less than a superhero. I had, after all, made it to graduate school and a rigorous career on my own. I never told a single professor or any employer about my health problems. I never asked for extensions or special treatment. In fact, I prided myself in my ability to make it on my own, and exposing this flaw seemed to me an admission of my limitations. I just could not bring myself to do that.

Life was going well. I was excited that I was going to be a therapist, I owned a house, and Taylor was going to start kindergarten in Barrington, Illinois, where I grew up.

Just after my thirtieth birthday I decided to try online dating with match.com to see if there were any special men out there. I knew that a man wasn't going to fall into my lap, and I also knew that I wanted to be married and for Taylor to have a father figure in the house. The first day on the site, I received a wink from a man named Joint Surgeon.

"What is a wink?" I replied. Match.com was working.

"I wanted to flirt with a pretty girl," he shot back.

I blushed at my computer when I read the word *pretty*. I was totally intrigued and excited to get to know Joint Surgeon.

"You think I'm attractive?" I wrote back.

"Yes. You got a wink, and I want to call you on the phone."

"No way!" I replied.

I wanted to get to know him a little longer than two minutes. I was not going to just give my phone number to a man I had just met on the Internet. He agreed to e-mail me for a bit longer so we could get to know one another, and I proceeded to ask him no less than a hundred questions—or at least I'm sure that is how it felt to him. I started with, "How many girls have you dated since your divorce?" I did not want to be his first date postdivorce. He clarified that I would not be, so I felt better about the flirting and about Joint Surgeon. We talked online every night for about a month, sometimes for hours and hours. I felt like I had fallen for him, and I had never even heard his voice!

I found out so much about this man named Shawn. He lived an hour and a half away from me a Chicago suburb called Beverly. He was a surgeon at a hospital in Chicago. He had also been through the wringer. He had lost his eighteen-month old baby and was raising his son, who had learning issues, alone. I told him about Taylor and about my last serious relationship, who of course was a doctor as well. Strange how the universe works. As we got to know each other more and more, he kept begging me to come meet him. Finally, I caved.

"I'll meet you at your office," I told him.

"Perfect," he said. "I want to show off my office anyway because it has beautiful views of the Lake Michigan."

I went to meet Dr. Shawn Palmer at his office with the beautiful views, and I was thoroughly impressed with both the man and the views. He had floor-to-ceiling windows that overlooked the entire city of Chicago and also Lake Michigan. I was so impressed; I had never seen Chicago from that vantage point. I was also baffled that a man like him had pleaded with me to meet him. I was leery of his enthusiasm, I guess. After all, don't they say everyone is dying to marry a doctor? That is what Dr. Organic always told me. That meant a doctor could get anyone they wanted, and it seemed Dr. Shawn Palmer wanted me. I wanted to be sure I didn't give in too easy, however, so I did not rush anything.

"Would you want to go out for lunch?" he asked.

"I suppose I have time," I told him.

During our first date, I asked him if he was dating anyone.

"Well, yes, kind of," he replied.

"Who is it?"

"Another doctor," he told me.

My question was out of curiosity rather than jealousy. I really didn't mind that he was dating someone. I figured we could just be friends because I really enjoyed talking to him. I was also getting used to my new house and was spread very thin, so dating someone who lived so far away would be a stretch. Taylor also had to see a tutor for help with reading, so I had plenty to keep me busy. I was also going to school and working for a developmentally disabled training center at a nearby school, so there was no time for Dr. Shawn Palmer. I really liked him, but I had limited time, and I was exhausted.

We said good-bye after lunch, and that night he called me and told me that he was no longer dating the doctor.

"Why?" I asked.

"Because I can't stop thinking about your brown pants," he replied.

"Why is that, Dr. Palmer? Why are you intrigued with my pants?" I asked playfully.

"I cannot tell you because I'm a gentleman," he quipped. And then he said it: "I'm falling in love with you. Our long conversations are beautiful, and I want to spend as much time together as possible."

Wow. I was not quite ready for that. I was not quite ready for anything, really. I just thought maybe I'd see what kind of men were out there. I hadn't imagined falling in love, especially so quickly.

"I'd like to see you again," he said. "And I'd like to meet Taylor the next time we meet. And you can meet Max."

I was blown away. As busy as I was, and as hesitant as I may have been about getting into a relationship with so much going on, I was compelled to say, "Yes!"

Dr. Shawn Palmer and Max arrived in Barrington in a brand-new Jaguar. He picked us up at my house and took us to a carnival. The children loved being together from the first moment. Neither of them had any reservations about the relationship. I, on the other hand, still had a few. I was afraid to be in a relationship, and for some reason my dad did not approve.

"You need time to yourself," he insisted. "You don't need men in your life right now. Finish graduate school, then worry about a man."

I usually took my dad's advice, but this time I decided to rebel a bit. I let myself enjoy our second date, and I loved seeing how much fun the kids were having together. The second date was a blended-family date, and it was going wonderfully.

After the carnival we went back to my house and had dinner, then soaked in the hot tub. I showed him what a fabulous cook I was—taking after my Grandma Catherine. I had been collecting recipes for years that both adults and kids would love. The entire night was a raging success. We planned for our next date—and our next after that. Max was turning five soon, so I planned his birthday party in my backyard. Fifty people came, and everyone loved it. This was the opportunity for everyone to meet my boyfriend, Shawn, and Max, his son. It was a success even though we did not have air conditioning in the ninety-degree Chicago summer. I showed Shawn the love of a family from the beginning. Togetherness and nurturing each other is what we have. We have had it from the very beginning.

I knew that despite my dad's feelings and my busy life that I wanted Shawn more than anything or anyone I had ever wanted, but wanting him also meant hiding something from him so I wouldn't ruin his view of me. Throughout our courtship, I never mentioned my pain or the symptoms I had been suffering since I was a child. For some reason, I was totally embarrassed at my bad health. I knew he wanted a strong woman after being alone as a single dad, so I wanted to be strong. I kept all my symptoms to myself so as not to burden him with them, and I married the man of my dreams in the Community of Church of Barrington in Barrington, Illinois.

Afterward, we went to Maui for our honeymoon. God planted the seed of a baby boy named Charles Edward Palmer. This was the start of our blended family growing to a family of five. Together, we had three children that are twenty-three months apart. I would get pregnant after Shawn touched me. Again, my symptoms would go away during pregnancy, and I would get pregnant again. Both Taylor and Max did not or rarely saw their biological parents. Here is my team, Team Palmer:

Taylor is twenty years old, and she is a chemical engineering major at the University of Iowa in Iowa City. Raising her as a single mother, I could not be any prouder. She dances to raise money for children with cancer. She is in a leadership position with her sorority, Kappa Kappa Gamma.

Max Palmer is my music maker who I'm very proud of. He loves to write music and is learning to drive.

Charles Edward Palmer, who Shawn and I call our Maui surprise, is identical to Shawn. He has a genius IQ, and Shawn and he travel together to South Africa every summer for a safari.

Sarah Mae Palmer, who has my favorite name ever, is the kindest child. Every time she smiles she lights up the room with her beautiful teeth and deep-green eyes just like her father. I call her my middle child with a pleaser personality. She reminds me of me when I was little, but she is another Shawn clone. She looks just like Shawn with long hair.

Finally, there is Katie Palmer. There is something about the youngest of five. She is stubborn like me. The apple does not fall far from the tree. She fights her way through everything and is sweet and special. I love her in every way.

I was on cloud nine, and I had kept my secret for thirty-one years, so I didn't see why I couldn't keep it my whole life. Secrets have ways of bubbling to the surface, however, and it isn't always up to us when we finally let them out. I may have been able to fight this mystery illness, but genetics can only be ignored for so long.

- 4 -

Never Say Never!

*I said I would never marry a physician after Dr. Organic,
but deep-green eyes drive me crazy, and he had a partner
named Max, who is perfect. Never say never in life.*

—*Melissa Mae Palmer*

At thirty-one, I married my soul mate, my rock, the love of my life. We brought our two children into our beautiful marriage and immediately began to grow our happy little family. Motherhood was always natural to me from the time I was a little girl playing with dollies and trying to help my mother with Billy. Because of my precious brother, I was ready and willing to become Max's mother—not his stepmother, but his mother. Both Shawn and I were also ready to add to our family immediately. I knew that I wanted a large family. At eleven years old, I could handle our entire household. My parents knew that dinner would be cooked and my brother and sister would be safe with me until they arrived home from work. I never saw taking care of them as a chore either. I loved being maternal to Billy and Mary. I couldn't wait to have my own children. As fate would have it, Shawn felt the very same way.

Blended families can work, but it can be a challenge. There were times that it was difficult because the children had to adjust to the marriage, but Shawn and I supported each other with parenting each other's child. We do a great job supporting each other and loving each child. Because of that, our blended family worked flawlessly, from dating, to marriage, to having three biological children together. We were one big happy family no matter what. There was always something lurking behind my picturesque family, however, and that was my secret—the illness I had been hiding my entire life. It stayed hidden until I could hide it no more.

Six years into our marriage, Shawn and I had welcomed two beautiful children into our lives. We thought we were finished, but it turned out we weren't. Right around Shawn's fortieth birthday, we found out about our little surprise. Shawn had scheduled a vasectomy the week I found out I was pregnant, so God surprised us with a fifth child! We could not be any happier. I was thirty-six, and Shawn was forty, and we were having our fifth little one.

The week before I found out that I was pregnant I had seen a rheumatologist in Chicago in an attempt to figure out what was going on with my body once again. I still had high liver enzymes and joint pain. I was diagnosed with Lyme disease; my diagnosis was the first case the doctor had ever seen. He put me on steroids, but I never filled the prescriptions because the next week I found out I was expecting. I didn't want to take steroids while I was pregnant. Strangely, I felt better than ever during the pregnancy, just as I had with the others. All the "Lyme disease" symptoms seemed to disappear as my pregnancy progressed. I had none of the symptoms that had plagued me for so long. After the first trimester, I had energy, my digestive tract was working well, and I felt no pain. I began to hope that whatever it was I had been suffering from my entire life had finally gone away—that I was miraculously cured. This was not the case. In fact, I would soon find out that there was no cure.

I had Katherine, or Katie, by way of cesarean after having to have an emergency cesarean with Sarah Mae. When I first saw her face, I was struck by how much she favored me. She could not have looked more like me. She was my little clone. I was thrilled, but after I had her, I had this bizarre bruising from head to toe. The bruising would unravel all my lies. It would expose me and show my husband that I was not the strong, untouchable woman I had always tried to be. It would be those bruises that would make me divulge everything—the pain, tiredness, diarrhea, and raging liver enzymes –that had been with me throughout my entire life. I was in love with him, and I wanted him to see me as perfect, pretty, and sexy. That is how I saw him, after all. And it is the way he always saw me too, even throughout my pregnancies and after being by my side as I gave birth to our children. I took pride in my looks and femininity. I loved looking beautiful for him, and I never wanted him to see what I considered the ugly side of me. I suppose I still had some lingering insecurities left over. I always wanted to excite him and turn him on. He was sure to let me know I did. He would tell me that I was absolutely exquisite. During my pregnancies, he made sure to let me know he saw me as gorgeous as ever. Every day he would rub my stomach and say how beautiful and sexy it was to have his baby inside of me.

"I hope the baby has big brown eyes with dark skin like you," he would say.

But just after Katie was born, we were about to hit rough waters that didn't allow for fairy tales or faultless beauty to remain enact. We were about to encounter a genetic mess that reminds all of us how human we all really are. I had been hiding fatigue and digestive issues for years, but that was all about to end. My mystery illness was creeping in deeper and deeper. The moment I hit my thirties, it began harder and harder to lie about it. I was getting new symptoms I couldn't hide like the others. People would ask, "Are you limping, Melissa?" I would brush it off and make an excuse because I was so embarrassed to be so young and limping. I found myself holding on to railings while climbing the stairs. I tried to hide everything by drinking a lot of coffee, going to sleep with the babies, and blaming limping on a sore back from holding the kids. I do not know how I was able to have four children in such a short amount of time, but I did. I also did all I could to hide that anything was wrong with me. I had to be perfect, so I pushed through the pain and continued to survive.

I needed to tell Shawn; I knew that. But his practice was picking up, and life was so busy. Because we went from strangers to intimacy with no friendship in between, I didn't know how to be vulnerable or real with him. I loved him so much, but I was afraid of dashing the image he had of me. I mean, how could I tell the man who works with orthopedic injuries all day that I have constant body pain? I figured he did not want to come home to complaints after hearing them all day from patients. Besides that, I had always taken care of myself and others. I did not want anyone to feel they needed to take care of me, and because of that, I never told him. To hide my other symptoms, I went on skipping meals so I wouldn't get sick. He thought I did it to stay thin, and so he didn't think twice about it. I often wondered if he would still love me if he ever found out that I was not this perfect wife. I was so afraid it would affect our relationship, and it did because I was always tired and weak but masking it. At the end of the day, the thing I had no name for was taking a toll on our marriage, and it left us with no togetherness. While I was able to avoid giving it a name for over four decades, the day finally came that I could no longer practice "What I don't know can't kill me" because I didn't know, but it was.

When I finally decided to come clean, I knew I needed to spill the beans to someone I truly trusted and someone who had known me my whole life. So when it all got to be too much to take on all alone, I went straight to my lifelong physician, a man named Dr. McDonough. He already knew that I was supposed to be seeing a hepatologist, also known as a liver specialist, because I had raging liver enzymes from the time I was nine. Since I had been going to see Dr. McDonough, however, I had never actually made an appointment with one. In fact, I had promised at least ten physicians over the last three decades that I would follow up with a liver specialist, but I didn't. If I saw a hepatologist, I would have to admit that there was something wrong with me, and I was not willing to do that.

I should say here, however, that there was nobody and nothing forcing me to hide my illness. Hiding everything and running away from it was my fault, and I do not recommend it to anybody. What I was essentially doing was putting off the inevitable as I suffered in silence. I had to find the strength to be diagnosed after a lifetime of sweeping all my symptoms under the rug. My entire existence was a little white lie at that point. The only other person outside of the doctors who knew anything was wrong was Jerry, who I told when we were going to Arizona State together. Besides him and the gastroenterologist in Phoenix, no one even knew I was in constant pain. I also had sensitivity to noise and diarrhea to the point that I was anorexic just to stave off the consequences of eating. The doctor just left it alone so I could conquer life and hide from it rather than face it. Sure, I had opportunities to tell others or go to a specialist, but I had so much to accomplish in my life before I could see a doctor. I let all the things to do distract me for decades, but finally, at thirty-six, I could hide no more.

- 5 -

A Secret Revealed

The mystery was not in my head. Finally, I can come clean with my symptoms.

—Melissa Mae Palmer

Shortly after I had Katie, the pain got so intense that I was collapsing pretty regularly. When it got to the point that I could not lift Katie, I decided enough was enough. The time was finally right to become my own advocate for my health. I made an appointment with Dr. McDonough, and with Katie in my arms, I walked into his office, ready to come clean.

"I have to get some kind of help," I told him. "The pain is just too much."

"Wow, Melissa. I've known you since you were a little girl. And I have never heard you complain about anything," he replied. "There's something wrong here, and we need to figure out what."

"I know," I said, fighting back tears.

"You are not the 'conquer the universe Melissa' I'm so used to. We're going to get you back to that," he assured me. "I don't want this to scare you at all, but you look weak and pale. I know as tough as you are that the only reason you're concerned is because it is affecting you as a mother. But don't worry. We're going to fix this, whatever it is."

Dr. McDonough was and is a huge champion in my life. He was a kind, caring doctor who was so popular that he could no longer accept any more patients. He helped bring my husband's job to Barrington in 2005 so he could be an orthopedic surgeon in my hometown. He had watched me grow up from the time I was just a child and then took care of my five children. As much as I trusted him, there was a part of me that was afraid he would misinterpret my symptoms as postpartum depression since Katie was only three months old, and that had happened to me before with Taylor Mae. I was afraid that he would say that everything was in my head or that my pain was subjective. I was also not terribly excited to tell my male physician that I had chronic diarrhea or that I was weak and could barely lift Katie to breastfeed her. My fear was that instead of taking my symptoms as health problems, the doctor would assume I was depressed and simply struggling with hormones, but he never did; he believed me from the beginning and started tests to find out what was causing so much pain for me.

"Did you ever follow up on those liver enzymes?" he asked me as he started drawing blood.

"No," I answered.

"Well, we know there is something wrong with you and we are going to get to the bottom of it. I'll take your lab samples, and I call you this week to let you know what we find out."

"Okay," I said softly as I waited for the blood to be drawn.

This doctor had known me my whole life; he'd been treating my family for generations. He was there for all my firsts, from my first set of stitches, my first-time experience "becoming a woman," and my first child. He knew everything about me—almost. The one thing he didn't know was about to be uncovered. He was about to discover the biggest mystery ever, not just about me, but for doctors everywhere.

"Melissa, I would like to see you and Shawn as soon as possible."

Those words spoke to me on the phone two days earlier by Dr. McDonough still echoed in my head as we sat in his office. Dr. McDonough had been my physician since I was twelve. Even with his boyish looks he always felt like a father figure to me. He was kind and gentle, always taking the time to listen as if nothing else mattered in the world. Over the years, his face has weathered slightly, and his dark hair has turned salt and pepper, but he still looks ten years younger than his age.

Dr. McDonough knew my liver had been erratic since I was a young girl. He hospitalized me twice: once in seventh grade and once when I was twenty-five. The first time was when I was suffering flu-like symptoms with elevated liver enzymes. The staff at the small community hospital were baffled at first. They believed I had toxic shock syndrome, something that can happen when girls wear tampons for too long of a time.

The second hospitalization came when I was in my early twenties. Taylor was just two years old. I had just arrived into O'Hare Airport from Arizona, where I was living. I was suffering from devastating diarrhea that would not stop and a high fever. By the time I got to Illinois I was severely dehydrated. I made a desperate call to my mother, who was working at Good Shepherd Hospital at the time. It was now the middle of the night, but she quickly arranged for me to be admitted. Once again, I had high liver enzymes.

The staff diagnosed me with food poisoning. Although Dr. McDonough was not completely convinced, I pleaded with him to let me go back home. Maybe he was just a softie, maybe he was tired of me begging—I'm not sure. He did release me with a prescription for a month of antibiotics. By the time I was finished with the antibiotics, I never felt better—at least for a while.

Later I would find out that Dr. McDonough had been suspicious of my condition for quite awhile. Unfortunately, I was so tight-lipped about my suffering—hiding it from everyone, including my parents, my friends, and, even now, my husband—he could never determine exactly what was wrong with me.

Just days before that fateful phone call from Dr. McDonough, I realized that I could no longer hold my secret in. Holding my three-month-old baby, Katie, in my arms, I felt as if my muscles were on fire. I was still bruised and sore from the C-section during her birth, but I was also very weak from my lifelong disease. I felt Katie start to slip through my grip. I quickly sat down and cradled my baby in my lap for support. The thought of how close I came to dropping her shook me to the core. I couldn't even hold my precious newborn in my arms. I had four other children to care for, two of which were young and expected their mommy to pick them up and hold them whenever they had a boo-boo or were frightened by a noise.

I sat there with Katie on my lap and wept. This secret that had been locked inside of me for all of these years could not be pushed back any more. I had fought it back all my life, but I was now too weak and exhausted to battle it any more. Yes, I hid and I ran away from these profound symptoms, but I could not any longer. I could not walk or lift Katie, my three-month-old, so I made an appointment to see Dr. McDonough, and, yes, I was so afraid to tell the truth finally.

Tall and lean, Dr. McDonough had a commanding presence when he walked into a room. With me, however, he was just my good-natured physician who always had a twinkle in his eye when he saw me. As I told him about my condition and how I had hidden it all these years, I felt his disappointment, although he did not show it. I know he was always there to help, wanting to assist me in any way he could, but I had never been able to bring myself to talk about it, even in the confidence of my doctor.

I felt ashamed that I couldn't trust him with my secret all these years. He had always been there for me. Dr. McDonough had even helped Shawn get a job when he lived in the city. Instead of making me feel bad, he quickly put me at ease and was only interested in finding out what was wrong with me. He ordered up a full batch of bloodwork and said he would get back to me as soon as the results came back.

"We'll get to the bottom of this, Melissa," he said assuredly. "I won't rest until we find out what's wrong."

Then came the phone call.

Now Shawn and I were sitting in Dr. McDonough's office on a Friday afternoon, waiting for him to enter. Shawn held my hand and was quiet. He was also pale, which was usually the case if he suspected bad news. Taylor was cheerleading for the high school football team that evening, and I was making small talk about the evening's plans when Dr. McDonough entered. I noticed immediately that the twinkle in his eye was gone. Instead, his eyes were watery. I felt a cold chill sweep through my body and my throat close off.

"Melissa, your CPK is really high," Dr. McDonough said softly.

I felt Shawn's hand tighten up, then relax quickly again, not wanting me to sense his concern.

"What?" I asked him, confused.

At that moment I didn't know what CPK meant, but Dr. McDonough and Shawn knew the seriousness of a high CPK.

"I need you to go down to Northwestern. I have no answers for you as of this moment, but there is a problem," he said, looking me straight into my eyes. "I want you to go as soon as you can."

The drive back home seemed to take forever. Shawn didn't say much as he drove, but I sensed his disappointment as well. My dark secret was finally coming out, a secret I felt too embarrassed to tell my loving husband. I could only imagine what he was thinking about.

As we neared our home, Shawn reached over and held my hand. "We'll get through this," he said. "I'll be there for you. I promise."

I soon would learn that CPK stands for creatine phosphokinase, an enzyme in the body. High CPK levels can indicate, among other things, muscular dystrophy, a disease that causes progressive weakness and loss of muscle mass, for which there is no cure.

What followed seemed like an endless array of tests that would finally unravel a lifelong mystery of what was plaguing me. During this journey I was poked and prodded so many times I began to feel like a human pincushion. There were times I wondered if all this grief and discomfort was worth it. I allowed these thoughts to flow into my mind, and like a stream, I let them flow back out. I knew deep within my heart that I needed to be strong for my family. It wasn't easy. I was never without doubt and fear, but I knew I was a survivor and that God had a plan for me.

At first, the Northwestern Health System thought it was a post-Lyme disease disorder because I had been bitten by a tick during a camping trip in Wisconsin. After that was dismissed, the muscular dystrophy department at Northwestern thought I had myotonic dystrophy, an awful disease that can be life-threatening. If it indeed was myotonic dystrophy, there was a good chance that our four children I'd given birth to may develop it as well.

It is one thing to be diagnosed with a disease that may eventually take your life. It is quite another to know that your precious children may inherit it from you. Our five children are vastly different from one another, but the one thing they have in common is that they are all very precious to Shawn and me. Taylor has grown into a beautiful woman. She is the head cheerleader at her school and excelled at everything she tried. Max has some obstacles he will always face and may never live alone, but he is perfect to us. Charles is strong like his father, although he does suffer from food allergies.

Sarah, on the other hand, had been the most difficult birth. At nineteen weeks, the doctors noticed she had only one functioning kidney. They were so worried that she wouldn't make it they gave me the chance to abort, but neither Shawn nor I gave it a second thought. We knew God would heal her. We wanted another child and prayed to God every night to let our baby be born alive. Sarah decided she was ready to come out into this world at thirty-two weeks, which resulted in a severe case of asthma until she was four. There were complications with her C-section, and I almost died, but someone was looking out for us both. Sarah is my miracle baby. At just two months she had surgery to repair her kidney, and she is now a happy, healthy child.

Lastly, Katie is the only child that looks like me. She inherited more than my looks though. She also inherited my strong will and independence, which makes for the occasional clash between mother and daughter.

I remembered my maternal grandmother, Catherine, originally from Czechoslovakia, and the ailments she suffered from. She complained of pain her entire life. Eventually she came to live with my Aunt Kathy, and I remember her staying on the couch during our visits. She was diagnosed with seronegative rheumatoid arthritis, but it was plain to see that something else was causing her pain. I believe that she had undiagnosed Pompe disease because my mother's side is so strong. When I asked why Grandma was in so much pain, the conversation would always change. We just didn't talk about anything bad and savored the fun family togetherness. Of course, I would grow up to perpetuate this family tradition. I hid from this illness and everything else my entire life. I hide from my problems. A lot of us do; it is a normal defense mechanism. It isn't just my illness that I avoid to keep the happiness in the family.

In 2002, Shawn lost his eighteen-month-old baby boy in an accident. He fell out of love with his wife at that time, but he stayed with her. Shawn spent most of his time alone and miserable. Shawn still doesn't like to talk about Sam, and I understand since I too have learned not to talk about the bad things. The children are sometimes curious about Sam, but when they ask, I simply say, "That makes Daddy and Max, our superheroes, sad. Let's not mention it or ask about it." The children idolize Shawn and Max, and they would never do anything to hurt them, so they always agree not to ask, but they are so curious about their brother. We took them to the cemetery once years ago and it was heartbreaking for Max and Shawn. Occasionally the other children will ask something about their brother, and I can immediately see beads of sweat line Shawn's forehead. I can only imagine the pain he suffers every day of his life due to that horrible event.

He had always wanted a big family and a loving spouse, something that he thought he'd never have, until he met me. Although I suspect he would prefer me to be a typical orthopedic surgeon's wife—one who does lunches, plays tennis, and socializes at dinner events—I am not that person. I love to socialize with others, but I prefer my true friends. When you have an illness, you find them. When I have the energy, my job is charity causes. I enjoy helping other people, and it makes me feel better. I prefer to keep busy with philanthropic events and writing media articles, though Shawn does seem to like it when fellow doctors approach him and say they have read his wife's work and praise the work she is doing for patients with illnesses. I support people with illnesses, and I always will. I majored in psychology because I have this innate desire to help others in any situation get better. Growing up, everyone always picked on my brother, and so I was always on the defense for him. I do not like to see the unemployed, underemployed, and ill being mistreated in this world. I volunteer in my free time to make this crazy universe better. No lunches or tennis for me; I'm sure not the typical surgeon's wife.

I am not a princess wife or a chronic patient. I am an advocate for our ill, a mother of five, and a loving wife. Shawn, I think, wishes that I would have lunches and more treats during the week, but I want to make a difference, and that is where my motivation lies. Shawn and I are hard workers from upbringing, and we teach our children to work hard and respect others. We tell them material goods are worthless and that it is love and respect that matters most. Shawn and I did not come from money; hard work is what gets you places in life.

Shawn and I are perfectly compatible in our desire to have a family. After we were married, God gave us our first child together, Charles. Charles is identical to Shawn in so many ways; both are handsome thin and strong. Charles is also a genius like his father. Their photographic memories astound me.

I enjoyed being pregnant because it was the only time that my symptoms went away— another medical mystery. Since I didn't have diarrhea, I could anything I wanted. I got to experience the joy of savoring food. Baked brie cheese with fruit on top was one of my favorites and so were jellies and baked potatoes with five kinds of cheese toppings. I was in food heaven. I did gain weight—

close to fifty pounds during each pregnancy—but I was always able to lose it afterward.

Another enjoyable aspect of being pregnant was having daily sex with Shawn. He loved the thought of his baby growing in my stomach. The weight gain didn't bother him in the least. His hunter instincts came out, and it made for some memorable nights. We were never closer than when I was carrying his precious babies.

It was these memories that kept swirling around in my head. If I did have this devastating disease, how could I bear the thought that my kids may one day get it too?

Once again I was back at Northwestern. This time I was meeting with a neuromuscular doctor, a lanky woman who spoke broken English. I will not use her real name here. Let's just call her Dr. Dread for reasons I'm sure you will eventually understand. As Dr. Dread sat down, she introduced herself without looking up at me.

"You have normal EMG," she said. "Abnormal blood work. CPK high and not going down. Muscle enzyme is in the 900s for last two months. Normal is in the 200s. Liver enzyme very high. Hips are extremely weak." She acted as if she were reading a grocery list rather than talking to a patient. In my mind, I thought how ironic it was for me to have weak hips when I was married to an orthopedic surgeon who specialized in joint replacement.

"Your genetic test came back negative for myotonic dystrophy," she said in an accent that was hard to comprehend.

"Wait, I don't have myotonic dystrophy?" I asked excitedly. She scared me. Shawn and I were so afraid for six weeks.

"That's what I said," Dr. Dread said dryly, completely cold to the fact that this was the best news I have heard in months. "You need a muscle biopsy. I have it scheduled in two days."

Two days just happened to fall on Christmas Eve. Being a procrastinator by trade, I wasn't ready for the Christmas holiday yet. There were still presents to buy, decorations to put up, and treats to bake. Plus, my mother was planning to move to Florida, and this would be the last holiday we would all be together.

"Can't we do this after Christmas?"

Dr. Dread shook her head. "You'll have your biopsy in two days."

"Okay then," I said, holding back my tongue. Secretly, I was ready to fire her ass as soon as the muscle biopsy was finished.

It was a cold wintery Christmas Eve when we drove to Northwestern University. Even though holidays are a busy time for surgeons, Shawn took the day off to be with me. As we drove past rows of houses with Christmas lights and decorations on their snow-covered lawns, I couldn't help think about the people inside. Many would be gathered around the fireplace, listening to Christmas songs and enjoying family traditions. At that moment, I envied them and hoped that I would live long enough to enjoy more Christmases with my family.

The walk to the neuromuscular department was a short one, but it left me chilled to the bone as the cold wind cut through my leather coat. I was shaking, and my teeth were chattering as we slowly warmed up in the waiting room. After about twenty minutes, we were led into an operating room, where we met Dr. Dread's partner. He seemed like the complete opposite of Dr. Dread. He was actually very warm and kind. Even though he was in a one-year residency and not as experienced as many, he had a caring personality, which made me feel at ease.

He gave me a numbing medication and started the procedure. Unfortunately, he had a hard time finding a sample. The biopsy lasted for three hours. He talked to me throughout the procedure and at least made the time go quicker. He talked about our children and how much they meant to us. Shawn was his usual quiet self, focused more on what the results might be than the procedure itself.

At one point I asked, "Can you be my doctor rather than Dr. Dread?" He laughed and said that he only does muscle biopsies and EMG reviews. Dr. Dread handles all subsets of muscular dystrophy. He did thank me for asking, and I admired him for not saying a single negative word about his partner. He told me that Dr. Dread would contact me with the results in four days, although I doubted she would be that prompt.

The biopsy left me bruised and sore. I put on the bravest face I could for the holidays, but the pain and weakness I felt was brutal.

I enjoyed the time with my family but secretly wanted to crawl into bed and stay there until I got the results back. Seeing the joy of my children with their new presents and enjoying their Christmas gave me temporary relief from the discomfort, but eventually the searing pain would rush over me.

Eleven days passed since the biopsy, and I still hadn't heard from Dr. Dread, so I called her office and left a message. When she called me back, she said I had holes in my muscle tissue.

"Holes? What does that mean?" I asked.

"It might be Pompe disease," she stated in her usual broken attempt at the English language.

The only Pompe I knew was this exquisite Italian restaurant in Chicago that was a favorite of Shawn and mine. Unfortunately, after being diagnosed with Pompe disease, I haven't eaten there again. No one wants to be reminded of a horrible chronic disease while they're trying to have a romantic dinner.

"I'm not a doctor, what is Pompe disease?" I asked her.

"Google it," was her unsympathetic response. "I advise you to call some doctors." I thought this was an odd remark since she was a doctor.

"What do you mean? Who should I call?"

"You need to call a pulmonary doctor and a cardiologist," she said then added, "and get a dried blood spot test."

Rudeness aside, I, at least, had my strongest lead yet. I had a friend who was a cardiologist in Barrington, so I immediately made an appointment with him and ran extensive tests. I then saw a pulmonary doctor, who made me do these awful lung tests that consisted of trying to blow up these balloons over and over. It was exhausting, and I could never do it adequately because of my disease. When the results came back, I had the breathing equivalent of a seventy-year-old man.

I also ordered a dried blood spot test, which is commonly used in gene screening. My results were drawn at Good Shepherd and came back with negative enzyme findings. My symptoms were indicative of Pompe disease but not of negative GAA findings. There is a mystery here about me, my symptoms, and my prognosis.

I also called Dr. McDonough, updated him on what was happening, and told him about my experiences with Dr. Dread. "I don't want to go back and see her ever again," I told him. He said he understood and vowed to get to the bottom of this. Since Dr. McDonough got the ball rolling in the first place, I was confident he would champion my cause. To this day, I believe he saved my life and will forever be grateful for his persistence and dedication to me and my family.

During this time, I did search the Internet for Pompe disease and learned as much as I could, just in case it was verified I did have it. Pompe is a rare disorder that is caused by the lack of the lysosomal enzyme alpha-glucosidase (GAA). The symptoms included muscle weakness, nausea, fatigue, and labored breathing—all of which I suffered from. It also said that Pompe can be potentially fatal. Was I already living on borrowed time?

Two days before my mother moved to Florida, Shawn, my mother, and I were in the car when Dr. Dread called me again. "The Mayo Clinic called me, and they confirmed you have no GAA. You do have Pompe."

It was finally official. At long last I knew for certain what was the cause of my lifelong suffering.

Later that day, Shawn locked himself in his office with strict orders not to be disturbed. He called every large hospital with a neuromuscular department. He was a man on a mission, and his love for me shone through brighter than ever. He was going to do everything he could to help me beat this disease. He finally found that Lurie Children's Hospital of Chicago had the Lumizyme replacement therapy that I would need as well as one of the best geneticists in Illinois. If I was approved, they could start me on an enzyme infusion every other week.

There was one thing I still had to do though. I had to call Dr. Dread and ask her to forward my report to Lurie Children's Hospital. I was nice and left a detailed message on her voice mail. It wasn't long before she called me back yelling, "You can't do anything with the muscle biopsy! We own it!" Dr. Dread wanted the tissue for research. Muscular dystrophy is a highly funded disease, and the tissue for a rare disease with profound scientific results could possibly change research funding for a hospital. These rare diseases bring in a lot of funding for large health systems. My muscle tissue at Northwestern meant that the hospital would receive the results and possibly get research funding.

It took everything within me to remain calm. "I'm sorry, but your lack of follow-up has caused me to go elsewhere. I cannot continue treatment with you," I said, feeling my face redden.

"If you want it, you will have to see me one more time!" The phone call ended abruptly.

I had no choice. I had to get the muscle biopsy report, so I drove out to Northwestern to see her. This time, however, Shawn came along. Dr. Dread's stance didn't surprise him. He told me that she wanted credit for diagnosing the woman with the profound rare disease. It could make her career. "We'll get the report," Shawn said confidently.

When we arrived in Dr. Dread's office, Shawn introduced himself. I could tell that Dr. Dread was intimidated by another doctor. Dr. Dread's attitude was vastly different. She even apologized for her previous behavior. She handed over the report without incident.

We walked out of the neuromuscular department, relieved that it went so well. "I knew we'd get the report," smirked Shawn. "But I had no idea we'd get it without a fight."

During our first trip to Lurie Children's Hospital, we met Shannon, a beautiful nurse practitioner who would champion our cause at the facility. She had possession of the precious muscle biopsy report and the dried blood spot results. She explained that because it was a children's hospital, she would have to get special permission from the board to treat me. The board was meeting the following week, and she acted like it wouldn't be a problem. I'm sure it wasn't as cut-and-dry as that, but with Shannon fighting for me, I knew our chances were good.

The following week I received a call from Shannon. She was elated to say that I was accepted and could start the enzyme infusions the next week. I was so happy tears rolled down my cheek. A long week of prayers had been answered.

The next few days were bittersweet for me. While I had a new lease on life with the treatments at Lurie Children's Hospital, it was also the week my mother left for Florida. We kissed. We hugged. We cried. I would miss her terribly. It broke my heart to see her leave, but a job in Florida was waiting for her, and I knew it was the right thing for her to do.

She needed to be with my father for their marriage, but I needed her. Divine intervention came into play. I had not progressed, and I had to be an adult. I wanted my mother to stay to be with me, but I had say good-bye to her and take care of myself.

On February 12, 2011, I said good-bye to my mother and hello to becoming a patient. It would be the start of seven years of enzyme infusions every other week at the Lurie Children's Hospital's oncology department. As time has rolled on, more doctors have become interested in my condition. GAA enzyme results reveal that any value under 40% is consistent with Late Onset Pompe Disease (LOPD). My value is 5.18%. To this day, the doctors who have studied my case cannot understand why I'm still alive and functioning. I have been called a genetic mystery. There were times in my life where I may have been skeptical of miracles. That is no longer the case. I'm living proof.

If you are reading this, please make sure to spend as much time with your kids, your spouse, your parents, and your friends as possible. Tell them you love them often. If you hold bitterness in your heart, please find a way to let it go. No matter how long you live on this earth, it is too short of a time. Only God knows how long we'll be here for. If we make the most of each day we're given and strive to make someone else's life a little better, we will have lived a life worth living.

My infusions are not easy to endure, and the road back has been difficult, painful, and humbling. There are times that I cry. There are times where I want to quit, but I pick myself up and find a way to carry on. I am still fighting the fight. I am still here for my devoted husband, and I'm blessed to watch my beautiful children grow. Every day I am thankful that I'm still here. I take nothing for granted. Believe me, I'm not that strong of a person. However, when I need that inner strength, it's there, and it pulls me through. If I can do it, then I know you can too.

We are survivors.

Learning About Pompe Disease

Pompe disease is a rare inherited neuromuscular disorder that causes progressive muscle weakness in people of all ages. The disease is named after Johannes C. Pompe, a Dutch doctor who first described the disorder in 1932 in an infant patient.[1] [2] However, Pompe can affect people of all ages, with symptoms first occurring at any time from infancy to adulthood.[1]

Pompe disease is caused by a defective gene that results in a deficiency of an enzyme, acid alpha-glucosidase (pronounced "AL-fa glue-CO-sih-days" and often abbreviated GAA). The absence of this enzyme results in excessive buildup of a substance called glycogen, a form of sugar that is stored in a specialized compartment of muscle cells throughout the body.

Disease Characteristics

The following pages in this section offer further details about Pompe disease, to help gain a deeper understanding of the underlying cause, progressive nature and classification of the disease.

- The underlying cause of Pompe disease is the same in all patients: a genetic defect causing deficiency of an important enzyme (acid alpha-glucosidase, GAA)
  Find out more about the cause of the disease

- The disorder is classified within several different disease categories, and doctors may refer to it by different names
  Learn more about classifying Pompe disease

- The progressive nature of the disease means that it always worsens over time, although the speed of this progression can vary from patient to patient
  Get more information on Pompe disease progression

- Genzyme offers printed materials to help better understand this rare and complex disorder
  Request educational materials

Pronouncing "Pompe"

There are different pronunciations for Pompe disease. In the United States, "pom-PAY" is typical, while in Europe it is usually pronounced "pomp-uh."

References

1. Hirschhorn, Rochelle and Arnold J. J. Reuser. Glycogen Storage Disease Type II: Acid Alpha-glucosidase (Acid Maltase) Deficiency. In: Scriver C, Beaudet A, Sly W, Valle D, editors. The Metabolic and Molecular Bases of Inherited Disease. 8th Edition. New York: McGraw-Hill, 2001. 3389-3420.

2. Pompe J-C. Over idiopatische hypertrophie van het hart. Ned Tijdscr Geneeskd 1932 76:304. No abstract available.

Getting Diagnosed

A complex and rare disorder, Pompe disease can be challenging to identify. Because of its progressive nature—it always worsens over time—it is important to diagnose Pompe disease as early as possible, so that appropriate patient care can begin promptly.

- One of the big challenges in diagnosing Pompe disease is that many of its symptoms are shared with other diseases
  Find out more about symptoms shared with other diseases

- Doctors use a variety of tests to investigate patients' symptoms, rule out other diseases, and arrive at a diagnosis
  Learn about the tests used for diagnosis

- Once suspected, doctors can use a blood test to quickly and simply screen for Pompe disease[1]
  Find out about tests to confirm a diagnosis

- As a genetic disorder, Pompe disease may also affect a patient's relatives, so other family members, especially siblings of an affected individual, may want to consider being tested
  Learn about genetic and family testing options

The Diagnostic Experience[2]

Getting diagnosed for Pompe disease can be a long and complicated process. It often involves several different doctors and a variety of tests, since symptoms may affect many areas of the body. Usually doctors need to first rule out other more common disorders that share similar symptoms with Pompe disease.

The experience is usually different for infants than for older patients because of the differences in how the disease affects these age groups.

Identifying the Disease in Infants[2]

Most infants with Pompe disease have severe symptoms that require immediate attention.

After seeing a physician, infants will usually undergo tests on their heart, lung, and muscles. An x-ray showing an enlarged heart—the characteristic sign of Pompe disease in infants—often alerts doctors to test for the disease.

Learn more about the signs and symptoms of Pompe disease in infants

Identifying the Disease in Children & Adults[2]

Among older patients, symptoms may emerge much more gradually and are not specific. It may take several visits, sometimes over months, before a confirmatory test is performed, especially if doctors are not familiar with Pompe disease. Often the combination of progressive (worsening) muscle weakness and breathing difficulties will alert doctors to test for the disease.

Learn more about the signs and symptoms of Pompe disease in children and adults

References

1. Winchester B, Bali D, Bodamer O, Caillaud C, Christensen E, Cooper A, et al. Methods for a prompt and reliable laboratory diagnosis of Pompe disease: report from an international consensus meeting. Mol Genet Metab 2008;93:275-81.

2. Kishnani PS, Steiner RD, Bali D et al. Pompe disease diagnosis and management guideline. Genet Med 2006 8:267-88.

genzyme

Pompe Fi

Patient Name: Melissa Palmer
DOB: 09/20/1973   Age: 37 yrs
SSN #:   Gender: Female

Genzyme Specimen #:
Case #:   Patient ID #:
Date Collected: 01/21/2011   Date Received: 01/26/2011

601354 / 312404

Chicago, IL 60611

Referring Physician:
Genetic Counselor:

Specimen Type: Peripheral Blood

Clinical Data: Suspected diagnosis

Client Lab ID #: F2/478
Hospital ID #:   102749029
Specimen ID #:
Specimen(s) Received: 2 - Lavender 5 ml round
                          bottom tube(s)

Ethnicity:

RESULTS: Sequence change detected ~ see below

DNA Sequence Change	Amino Acid Change	Classification	Note
c.-32-13T>G (heterozygous)	N/A - splice site	Clinically significant	See Interpretation & Comments
c.742delC (heterozygous)	p.L248fs	Clinically significant	See Interpretation & Comments

INTERPRETATION:

This analysis identified two clinically significant sequence changes, which are expected to cause Pompe disease when they occur on different chromosomes. Therefore, parental samples are required to determine whether these changes occur on the same or different chromosomes.

COMMENTS:

c.-32-13T>G is a mutation known to be clinically significant (e.g. Laforet P, et al. Neurology 2000; 55:1122-1128, Kroos MA, et al. Neurology 2007; 68:110-115).

c.742delC (p.L248fs) is clinically significant based on a predicted change in the protein.

The following sequence changes were identified in this specimen. Individually, each of these sequence changes is currently not known to be causative of Pompe disease. If these changes are found in a high-risk individual, identified by enzyme screening, biopsy or further clinical follow-up is recommended.
  Homozygous (two copies): c.1581A>G (p.R527R)
  Heterozygous (one copy): c.324C>T (p.C108C), c.547-4C>G, c.596G>A (p.R199H), c.642C>T (p.S214S), c.668A>G (p.H223R), c.1203A>G (p.Q401Q), c.2133A>G (p.T711T), c.2338A>G (p.I780V), c.2553A>G (p.G851G)

The above interpretation is based on the clinical information provided and the current understanding of the molecular genetics of Pompe disease. The Pompe full sequencing assay is expected to detect >99% of previously reported Pompe mutations. This analysis cannot rule out the presence of large deletion or duplication mutations, complex rearrangements or mutations in regions not analyzed.

Consultation with a physician or genetic counselor is recommended to discuss the potential clinical and/or reproductive implications of this result, as well as recommendations for testing other family members.

METHOD/LIMITATIONS:
DNA is isolated and amplified by the polymerase chain reaction (PCR). The entire coding region (exons 2-20) of the GAA gene and flanking intronic sequences (15 base pairs upstream and 5 base pairs downstream of each exon) as well as 32bp of UTR for exon 2, 30bp of UTR for exon 20, and portions of IVS17 and IVS18 (to detect the exon 18 deletion), are analyzed by bi-directional direct DNA sequencing using capillary gel electrophoresis and fluorescence detection. Clinical significance is predicted using information derived from the scientific literature, the Pompe Center mutation database, and tools such as SIFT and PolyPhen. False positive or negative results may occur for reasons that include genetic variants, blood transfusions, bone marrow transplantation, erroneous representation of family relationships or contamination of a fetal sample with maternal cells.
REFERENCES:
PubMed
PolyPhen: http://genetics.bwh.harvard.edu/pph/
SIFT: http://blocks.fhcrc.org/sift/SIFT.html
Pompe Database: www.pompecenter.nl

Electronically Signed by:
Reported by: 7KK

Testing performed at Genzyme Genetics 3400 Computer Drive, Westborough, MA 01581 1-800-255-7357   Page 1 of 2

genzyme

Pompe F

Patient Name: Melissa Palmer
DOB: 09/20/1973   Age: 37 yrs
SSN #:   Gender: Female

Genzyme Specimen #:
Case #:   Patient ID #:
Date Collected: 01/21/2011   Date Received: 01/26/2011

Referring Physician: Client Lab ID #:
Genetic Counselor: Hospital ID #:
                                  Specimen ID #:
Specimen Type: Peripheral Blood Specimen(s) Received: 2 - Lavender 5 ml round
                                                        bottom tube(s)
Clinical Data: Suspected diagnosis   Ethnicity:

601354 / 312404

Chicago, IL 60611

The test was developed and its performance characteristics have been determined by Genzyme The laboratory is regulated under the Clinical Laboratory
Improvement Amendments of 1988 (CLIA) as qualified to perform high complexity clinical testing This test must be used in conjunction with clinical
assessment, when available.

Electronically Signed by: Lynne S. Rosenblum, Ph.D., FACMG, on 02/08/2011
Reported by: /kk

Testing performed at Genzyme Genetics 3400 Computer Drive, Westborough, MA 01581 1-800-255-7357   Page 2 of 2

Neuromuscular Laboratory

                                          Director
                                          , Clinical Consultant
                                          Clinical Consultant
Chicago, IL 60611   , M.D., Clinical Consultant
Phone   Clinical Consultant
FAX (3   M.S., Supervisor

Muscle Biopsy Report

Patient Name: Melissa Palmer   **Referring Physician:**
Biopsy Number:
Biopsy Date: 12/13/10   **Biopsy Site:** left quadriceps
D.O.B.: 09/20/1973   **Clinical Diagnosis:** Muscle weakness
NMH MR#:

Gross Description: The specimen was of adequate size and preparation.

Microscopic Description: The H&E and modified Trichrome stains showed a significant variability of fiber size. A large number of fibers had vacuoles filled with basophilic material. These vacuoles were either subsarcolemal or central, some fibers had many vacuoles, and some vacuoles extended throughout the length of the fiber on longitudinal cuts. Nuclear clumps were scattered throughout the biopsy. Both the perimysial and the endomysial connective tissue were increased. No clear necrotic fibers were present but many fibers had a ghost like appearance. No regenerating fibers were noted. Active inflammatory changes were not appreciated. The intramuscular blood vessels were normal. The NADH-TR stain highlighted the significantly disturbed intermyofibrillary network. No dark angular fibers were seen. The modified Trichrome staining highlighted the vacuolar changes as described above and did not reveal any nemaline rods or ragged red fibers. The ATPase series at three pHs showed a normal mosaic pattern of fiber types. The vacuolar changes affected type 1 fibers predominantly. Acid phosphatase activity was significantly increased in many fibers and in some of the vacuoles. The PAS staining showed an increased staining in certain fibers and in some of the vacuoles; this excessive staining resolved when amylase was added confirming its glycogen nature. The non specific esterase showed no denervated fibers.

The Sudan black, myophosphorylase, AMPDA, VVG, cytochrome oxidase, SDH and alkaline phosphatase stains added no additional information.

Impression: This is a significantly abnormal muscle biopsy. The changes as described above are indicative of a vacuolar myopathy, and in particular of a glycogen storage disorder.

Assistant Professor, Neurology

01-24-2011
Date

- 6 -

Solving the Mystery

Survivorship—when you're down, find someone who will bring you up such as a partner. The pain was never in my head, as most people are told. This mystery was solved.

—*Melissa Mae Palmer*

I do not know how I spent two years alone at Lurie Children's Hospital in the oncology Department with the children receiving chemotherapy, but I did it. The nicest staff works at Lurie Children's Hospital, which is good because we made a family decision to keep my diagnosis quiet, so no one came to visit me while I did infusions. I spent my six-hour infusions talking to the parents who were with their children getting chemotherapy.

Because of the treatments, my Pompe stopped progressing. Still, it was a time-consuming affair. I sat in a small infusion room with children getting chemotherapy and vomiting everywhere. I would reach out the parents of the children and listen to their heartbreaking stories about their ill children or their dwindling finances, and I would try to help them in any way I could. I told myself that I had it so much better because even if I was sick, I got to go home to these healthy children of mine. Seeing those beautiful children getting those awful cancer treatments put my life into perspective. We all are survivors, and even though I'm a chronic patient, I have healthy, gorgeous kids. I realized that even more as I saw those innocent little ones getting chemo. My heart broke for the parents I got to know, and I got to know them well because they were the only people there I talked to because I never told anyone I was there. That was my way to deal with it—alone.

Shannon would stop by every treatment and to check in on me. She was incredibly nice. Even with her, however, it was lonely, and I rarely saw adults. That is, until one day when my favorite RN came in and said, "There is a man that is your same age who is getting treatment for Pompe disease." I went to meet this man, who had the same illness as I did; he would be the first Pompe patient I would meet.

It was nice to finally meet adults. Through chatting we found out that we lived in opposite ends of Chicago. As we were talking, it occurred to me that there had to be a way to transfer to Barrington, Illinois, at Good Shepherd Hospital. I asked Dr. McDonough, and he said he would look into it. He met with the Genzyme sales representative and took a class to learn more. Again, he did so much work to help me.

Good Shepherd approved me, and so finally I was coming home. The transition was seamless. I said my good-byes to Lurie Children's and left. I was so excited to go home to get my treatments, but still I left that day sobbing. I had met some amazing people. As sad as I was, however, I was elated to be close to home. I would be close to my children and only have a short drive if there was an emergency at home. Lastly, I would be with adults in the oncology department. I already had a friend named Debbie Overton who worked in the department.

Treatment days meant a full day at the local community hospital getting infusion with a bunch of nurses running around and checking on me every thirty minutes because I once had a severe reaction to the medication. My heart rate skyrocketed one day, so they changed my infusions and watched me like I was a ticking time bomb. What is a little blessing in disguise is that I was very familiar with the hospital I spent so much time in. My mother once worked as a full-time RN at the same hospital to support our family, and there I was as an adult getting the most expensive treatments in the universe to fight for survival. Life works in funny ways.

I would forget about the intense hospital day when I would go home to my children and lie on the most comfortable couch. I would look at my dream man and just be grateful. The next day, I was a normal mother again, just sicker from the treatments. Shawn would make dinner, and we would play with our children all night until I passed out from all of the medications I received during the infusion. It would make me so tired I felt like I was in outer space, but I wasn't. I was at home, where I belonged.

The best secret of survivorship I can give anyone is to look at your children and your spouse, think of things that bring you happiness, and move on. You cannot change anything in life, and I have learned that, but you sure can appreciate your blessings and move forward. With this attitude, I have been able to take my series of health issues as opportunities to become stronger. Most importantly, I had a wonderful husband, beautiful children, and a life I wouldn't trade for anything in the world. How could I ever decide that is not worth fighting for? Something I learned as I struggled through graduate school was how to forget about anything that is bothering you and to cope with challenges. I found some are not as healthy as others, however. Repression, for example, is something I used often that was probably a defense mechanism. I used it to block my feelings unconsciously, but then I learned to be open, honest, and free. I have found that life is filled with little surprises, both good and bad, and the only control we have is how we react to them. I chose to handle all that life hands me with an attitude of appreciation for all I have.

My family, friends, champions, and physicians have all told me that my attitude and motivation to live my life and fight have been what separates me from all other Pompe patients. I can't argue. I suppose I am, after all, a rarity in the truest sense. I'm fighting a severe case of a disease that should leave me paralyzed, but here I am, walking and breathing. According to the top doctors who study my disease, that just does not make sense. I have next to no natural enzymes. My blessings are keeping me alive with enough enzymes for a dead person. It's divine intervention.

Below are some of my test results that help explain, or expose, a little about my mystery illness.

- 7 -

Becoming an Advocate

I'm sick of Pompe. Do I really need treatment
after six years?

—*Melissa Mae Palmer*

S hawn and I decided to come out with our secret called Pompe
disease in 2013. I contacted my friend Chrissie Mena, who
owns a local media company, and my physicians to discuss this
decision and how to approach it. At the time, I had ten physicians.
We decided to bring awareness to this rare illnesses.

Meeting Chrissie Mena is 2005 was so interesting and
inspirational to me in so many different ways to my life as a mother,
wife, and a person. We immediately had this amazing connection.
I had learned that she had her media business with a background
in leadership of charitable organization and marketing. Now, eight
years later, she owns a highly successful media entity in Barrington,
Illinois. She is quite a blessing to me. She was an inspiration to
me because she was involved in a lot of charities, including Good
Shepherd Hospital, at the time we met, but we were at different
stages in our lives. I was getting married, and she was raising twin

daughters as well as an older beautiful daughter. She is a decade older than I am, and our relationship has become one of sisters. I have a decade plus to learn from her as a mentor and a champion. We have accomplished amazing things together even as we have always been at different life stages. Being a mother of older children while having babies and being a new wife to Shawn, for example, was difficult for me. In 2006, I was not able to be on the local auxiliary with her when I wanted to, but we have still always found ways to work together.

At the end of the day now she's a champion and an amazing friend to me. In 2013, Shawn and I decided to come clean about Pompe disease, and who did I call? Mrs. Chrissie Mena. I ran into her and told her that I had this rare disease called Pompe disease, and I wanted her to do a story on me because she is an amazing community leader and also owns a media website that is successful. She is gala chair of JourneyCare and has been president of a number of organizations, including GSH Auxiliary, BJWC, and BAUW. Every surgeon wanted the story about me with Pompe disease, and so did my team of ten physicians, so I asked Chrissie if I should invite the media to a treatment of mine and also if she would write a story on Pompe disease. She said yes. I wanted her there and to have ownership of the story. All of my treating physicians were there, and Chrissie spearheaded it and led it all. The whole interview was to build awareness on genetic illnesses and local residents affected by them.

Together we decided to discuss my rare disease and my experimental biweekly Lumizyme treatment. We worked with Good Shepherd Hospital and invited the *Daily Herald*, *Chicago Tribune*, and *Suburban* press. The day I was to make my disease public was picking up a lot of press. I also asked my team of doctors to show up at 1:00 p.m. Chrissie managed them; they all were there to support me. I get terrible anxiety with crowds, so my heart started to race as I fielded questions about Pompe disease, my symptoms, and the cost of the medication Lumizyme. I was scared because no one knew that for the past two years I had been travelling to Lurie Children's to get my medication so

I could live and receive acid maltase. My heart raced, and I felt some pressure because I was the focus. Chrissie cared about me and not just my story. She acted as a friend, not as the owner of a media business that day, and kicked them out with the head nurse, Donna. After we kicked the media out she stayed with me until I calmed myself down. We became inseparable. Chrissie took an interest in the global issue surrounding genetic illnesses and the research surrounding cures for genetic illnesses. She followed me through this voyage and has taken me to Duke to meet the world's leading geneticist. Since then I have received requests to do follow-up articles, and I have declined.

Chrissie is kind; she is the type of friend that when I'm sick I can ask for grape popsicles and she will take time to drop them off even though she is a successful mother of three, a wife of twenty-eight years, and the CEO of her own business. She takes care of me when I need her. I rarely ask anyone to do anything for me because I prefer to take ownership of my life in every way, but if I really need something, she is available; she is always ready to help out. She has been a good friend to me, and I look up to her. She runs the community with her philanthropy work and has three gorgeous daughters and a husband who is pure talent in marketing. We are so different, but we want answers about Pompe, and we are searching for them.

From Chrissie's Perspective

I first met Melissa Mae Palmer in 2005. At a party of mostly women, she approached me.

"I heard you are involved at Good Shepherd Hospital," she said. "I want to help."

I was the president of the hospital auxiliary at the time. It was a mostly older crowd, so I was thrilled that someone younger was interested in joining us.

Newly married to an orthopedic surgeon, she shared that she had also been a medical products representative. She explained that her husband would soon be practicing in the area, and she wanted to do what she could to help support the local medical community. We agreed to get each other's contact information from friends.

Being two women with busy lives and families, we did not get each other's information. I did run into Melissa a few times over the next couple of years; each time she was pregnant. I joked that we would get together when she stopped having babies. Melissa was always gregarious and completely charming. I looked forward to eventually working with her on charitable pursuits.

Unfortunately, a few years passed by, and when I ran into her again, she did not look the same. We were at the local high school football game. I had started a local media company and was covering the event. Melissa was there for her daughter Taylor, a varsity cheerleader. After greeting each other Melissa said, "I don't know if you heard, but I am sick."

She explained that she had Pompe disease and described what she had been through before she was finally properly diagnosed. She had recently moved her treatments to our local hospital, so I asked her if I could come and learn more from her doctors and caregivers.

The more I researched Pompe disease, the more my admiration for Melissa grew. I learned that Pompe disease is a rare genetic inherited neuromuscular disorder. The symptoms of the disease cause muscle fatigue, making simple daily tasks like getting out of bed and doing household chores very difficult. At the hospital I learned that the medication she was receiving was administered every other week and took up to six hours. She receives a drug called Lumizyme intravenously. The drug replaces an enzyme missing in patients with Pompe disease. The process looked painful, but Melissa was all smiles and compliments.

"I am so lucky," Melissa said as she was hooked up to the medication drip with monitors tracking all of her vitals. "Dr. McDonough did not give up on me. He pushed to find out what was really wrong with me."

Dr. McDonough also had approached Advocate Good Shepherd Hospital to administer Melissa's Lumizyme treatments.

Previously, she had to go down to Lurie Children's Hospital in the city of Chicago for treatments. With travel time, that meant she was far away from her young family for an entire day. Having the treatment locally allowed her to be close to home and to be there for her children as much as she could.

The disease has also made it necessary that she see many medical specialists. Because her muscles are weakening, she needs to see an orthopedic specialist regularly. She also sees a cardiologist to make sure her heart is not damaged. Most importantly, she sees a pain specialist regularly to help with the ongoing, sometimes crippling, pain she experiences. I tagged along to appointments with her pain specialist Dr. Tim Lubenow at Rush University Hospital on a few occasions. Tim was amazed at Melissa's attitude and credited her will as one of the reasons she would remain active and lead a productive life.

"It is so hard to see people give into the pain," Dr. Lubenow shared with me. "So many of my patients give up and end up in wheelchairs before they need to. Melissa pushes through. I wish all my patients had her determination."

Learning more about Melissa and her challenges, I realized what a truly unique person she is and how she refused to let herself be defined by her illness. I had never really thought about it in the past. Many people I had known, some diagnosed with diseases far less challenging, became victims to their disease.

Melissa and I became close friends over the next few years. Most of the time I forget that she had an illness because she is so positive and willing to be part of life's adventures. We both had big challenges we had to face more recently. I lost my brother suddenly from a heart attack, lost my brother-in-law in a car accident, and lost my father from a burst aneurism. While I was dealing with my family, Melissa had a life-changing surprise. In typical Melissa style, she met the diagnosis head on and scheduled surgery and treatments immediately.

I accompanied her to Duke University to see Pompe expert Dr. Priya Kishani. Melissa had been traveling to see Dr. Kishani annually for a few years. On this trip, during some routine exercises, Melissa's pain overwhelmed her. She pushed herself so hard physically her body finally fought back. The frustration was clear, and tears streamed down her cheeks. When her tests were finished, we met with Dr. Kishani, who revealed that many of those physical test results were better than years past. Although Pompe disease is progressive and eventually fatal, Melissa, by sheer will and determination, is going to put up the best fight.

Sharing a hotel room I wondered aloud, "If you continue to fight Pompe disease and not give into it—and continue to communicate and champion for people to understand what it is—you could help find a cure."

Melissa doesn't realize how unusual she is. She just wakes up and tackles every day, making the most of everything that comes her way. I am lucky to call her friend and am convinced that through her tenacity, she will be a part of finding a cure. At the very least, Melissa will lead people, by example, to live life to the fullest, no matter their illness and diagnosis.

Chrissie was really interested in learning about rare diseases and the treatments, and so was I. As time progressed, I thought that I should learn more about Pompe disease, and that is how I found Duke University. It is the leader of research. I connected with the head genetic physician Dr. Priya Kishani. Once we were in contact with her, my friend and I asked her countless questions about Pompe disease. We also went out to dinner with the other patients. They were all so welcoming and easy to talk to.

I was learning more and more about my disease, but at home with the family we pretended as I was normal. The fact was, however, I was not, and I was feeling pretty bad. I decided to reevaluate my results again, but I could not move my neck. The scoliosis that I had as a child had caused severe back pain. When I had the imaging studies done, they showed I had eight disks that were herniated in my spine. Life was in the way again. I decided to go see Dr. Chow at Rush University. We decided on a single-neck fusion, and with that I decided to look up my friend and expert Dr. Tim Lubenow.

Around this time my husband asked me to go off of treatment for the disease so I wouldn't be in the hospital so much. I had a special friend at Good Shepherd named Deb Overton, who has taken care of me like I'm royalty for over two decades, who I adored seeing, but the treatments were invasive, and I was sick the entire day after them. I love seeing her, but having side effects for two out of fourteen days is difficult with the demands of a family. I also did not want to be on medication and was also sick of the side effects. I decided to explore it more, which led to even more discoveries. I found out that I have close to no acid maltase, along with other interesting tidbits that sometimes lead to more questions, but I am convinced we will find the answers someday.

I have learned more and more about my disease over the years, but there is still so much work to be done within science to figure both Pompe and my personal genetic code out. Mine is the first living genetic code seen other than a male in medical literature from 1950, and it was identified by the University of Florida and Duke University. No one knows what that means with my case. I have one of the rarest diseases with the rarest genetic code. I am doubly rare and doubly perplexing to doctors.

With Pompe disease, you are measured from a scale of 1–40. In 2016 I found out that I come in at a five. I was shocked, and so was my husband. I make next to nothing of an enzyme called acid maltase—it is required for the body to function and for life to go on. Universities love my tissue for research studies, and I'm willing to help others with my results. I'm a lab rat for three reasons: one, I have the first genetic code with such a profound illness; two, my muscle biopsy was severe; and, three, my body does need a lot of acid maltase. I will do anything for scientific research to help figure this out, so I chose the best qualified doctor at Duke to analyze my very unique genetic code.

I have a chronic illness and one of the most severe cases ever recorded. I have a unique genetic code, the most unique to mankind. What does that mean? We do not know yet, but I believe some day we will. I have the only genetic code seen since 1950 in man from the Netherlands, but there is no information about his outcome. I am science's next shot at regaining that lost information. When I think about that man—a stranger I will never know—I always wonder how long he lived and if he fought. In the end, it does not matter, however, because I'm different, and I'm positive. I'm different from the other patients who have this same illness because I can walk and go on a rowboat. I see this not just as resilience but also as divine intervention. That is me. God is looking out for me, but I am fighting along the way. I will wait and see where else He will take me. Maybe God gave me another genetic mutation to protect me that they have yet to find, or maybe he sent me along so doctors could finally figure something out about this illness. Whatever it is, I know that good will come from my pain and that my unique circumstances will shed light where there has been none. As we work to identify this scientific mystery that my symptoms are not as profound as others while my bloodwork is more severe, I will also work to help others learn to survive.

We have gotten some strange answers this year that we are trying to make sense of for the people with this illness. Duke University found from doing skin fibroblasts that I have low levels of a certain essential enzyme for basic survival called acid malaise. That makes my illness all the more perplexing. Is my life divine intervention for our Lord or simply science? Perhaps it is both. One thing I know for sure is that is has been a geneticist's fight.

This mysterious illness that I hid my entire life is confusing, even to the top geneticist physicians in the world. Why am I so different than the other people with Pompe disease? My Pompe friends are all different; they all have varying degrees of pain and paralysis. Some have heart troubles; some have lost mobility. I feel so badly for my Pompe sisters and brothers because most of them are in walkers and have severe breathing problems. It is tough to say why we are all so different because there isn't a lot of scientific information about the disease. I have this pain that I have felt my entire life that was undiagnosed, and I realize that there are so many others that may have the same thing and do not know. I can't help but wonder if my beloved grandmother actually had Pompe. We have found that the genetic code I have that causes it comes from my mother's side. I do not think it is a coincidence that my maternal grandmother spent decades of her life in a wheelchair with no answers, but perhaps I have finally found her answer.

The genetic code I have could have been completely debilitating the way it was from my own grandmother, but it is not. It is in the infantile genetic code, and my case in particular is extremely rare and incompatible with life, but I am still out paddleboarding with my children. I never understood science, so this is a learning game for me. I rely on my husband to explain things to me since he is a medical doctor and I deal in the lexis of psychology for my own work. What I know well is that life has brought challenges for me from the time I was a child, and this disease began taking its toll on me at an early age, but I have found that I do have some control in my life still. I get to choose how I look at my situation, and I make the best out of everything, and I found survivorship. Every trying situation that I have been through I have fought for survival, and I have won. It is time to move on and only focus on the positives because it is in God's hands. How do I do this? We can't change the imminent, but we can find joy with our blessings. That is how I believe I am walking, breathing, and excelling at life when every doctor and scientist can see I should be in a wheelchair. I have had my fair share of surprises, to be sure. During each diagnosis, I have said to myself that I'm going to win, I'm going to beat this. I have survived because I know my life's purpose is to do just that so I can be there for my children, husband, and family.

As I think about the anomaly that is my life, I tend to ask myself what it is about me that has made me so very different. Why, I wonder, am I thriving when it doesn't make scientific sense? My Pompe test results are profound. I ask myself if it is my mind or science that is keeping me going. I have come to the conclusion that it is my mind because I have survived over and over again. In life you need to fight to get what you want, and that is exactly what I have done since I have been a little girl. For now, I'm healthy and normal. Each illness was severe, and I know that Shawn had no idea that his wife would have so many health scares so early in life, but we have made it through everything masterfully because of our outlook. He has done an amazing job dealing with it. He deals with sick people every day, and to have to deal with sickness in such a personal way was a shock at first, but now we are used to everything. Now he is my cheerleader; he tells me to beat Pompe like I have everything else in life.

It helps to believe in God and to have a solid support system at home that is loaded with family, champions, and friends. This is the philosophy of my foundation and what I tell others that are newly diagnosed with any life-threatening illness. People really need to hear this when they have seen a doctor for the first time and do not know what is wrong. My advice is to lean on your support system during testing and doctor visits because it will make everything in your life much easier. When things have been tough for me—and they certainly have been at times—my first move is to lean on friends and family. With love and championship, one can overcome some of the greatest obstacles in life.

God gave us our blessings and our challenges, but my blessings definitely outweigh the challenges. My life is about survivorship and winning the fight while dealing with those challenges. It has been our journey. All I can do now is think about the fact that God's love is infinite. My life has been colorful and unique to say the least. I have experienced so much, and I have always come out on top by fighting. There are times I want a break from fighting to enjoy the simple pleasures in life, like the sun and being a wife and a mother—one without pain—but I work around it. I do have choices: one is to enjoy life, and the other is to sit in a chair like my grandma. I'm going to enjoy every second on earth and be happy.

Survivors of anything, please let anyone know of symptoms or if anything is wrong because suffering in silence is no way to live a happy life. It is a good tip to keep your list of close people small because they have stayed with me through situation after situation. With five children, it has been important. These people have helped me with the carpools and children, and they sincerely ask me, "How are you feeling?"

- 8 -

From a Mother's Perspective
by Nancy Mae D'Agostin,
Who I Love So Much

September 20, 1973, at 4:35 p.m., God blessed us with a beautiful baby girl. We named her Melissa Mae, and she was perfect. She weighed seven pounds, two ounces and had dark hair, long dark eyelashes, and rosy cheeks. She had a sweet spirit, and we adored her.

She grew and developed normally and had a wonderful, happy personality. We took her everywhere, and she was so well behaved that we were always proud of her.

She loved to be around people and was very comfortable in a social setting. We took her to her dad's business shows, and she acted more mature than some of the adults. (She was only five years old.) From ages 5–12 she was active in school activities: brownies, softball, and boating. She had a lot of friends and was kind to everyone. Her brother was born when she was three and a half, and her sister arrived when she was five years old. She enjoyed her siblings and was definitely the leader of the "pack!" She was gentle yet firm with them, and I believe that this is when she practiced her mothering skills. Did I mention that she is an awesome mother?

Melissa was slender as a child and was somewhat of a picky eater. She loved eggs, and I was relieved that she ate this complete protein. Also, she liked fruit, veggies, creamy dishes (chips and dips), and filet mignon. She was most fond of Italian and Czech food, which her grandmas cooked with the authenticity of their respective heritages. She was not a sickly child by any means. She was, however, petite, and I worried about her losing weight when and if she got sick.

Our family moved from Hinckley, Ohio, to Barrington, Illinois, when Melissa started junior high. Her dad was transferred with his job, and in some ways we felt like we were going home. We still had family in the Chicago area, and that was good. Of our three children, the move was the most difficult for Melissa because she had to leave her friends from grade school. In a short time, however, she did meet new friends with whom she remains friends to this day. These friends have been a tremendous support to her as she has gone through some serious health issues. What is the saying? "You can never have enough friends."

When Melissa started high school she continued to meet new friends and was very active. During this time, she went to Mexico for a short exchange program sponsored by the Spanish department. She stayed with a wonderful family who had a son named Jose. The family was so impressed with Melissa that they requested that Jose stay with us when he was an exchange student in the USA. He stayed with us for a semester, and we learned about his culture. He and Melissa both joined the swim team during this time. Melissa was a great swimmer and also enjoyed roller boarding. She would take the dog out with her while roller boarding, and the dog would come back panting. She, however, was fine after the exercise. Nevertheless, the dog loved going running with her.

During her high school years is when she talked about experiencing abdominal discomfort and diarrhea. She went to the doctor for these symptoms and was diagnosed with endometriosis.

According to the doctor this was a fairly common diagnosis for suburban high school girls. Our plan was to monitor her symptoms unless they became worse.

After high school, Melissa went to college and received her degree in psychology. We were very proud of her accomplishments. Upon finishing college, Melissa met a charismatic man named Mark. They were married and had a beautiful wedding. It was a joyful celebration in which our families delighted. As Melissa started her professional career she worked as a sales rep for an endoscopy company. She excelled in sales, and we teased her that she inherited her dad's friendly, sincere personality, which allowed him much success in sales. She kept up a fast pace during this time period and was successful. She was also successful in giving us an amazing granddaughter named Taylor Mae. Taylor was our precious angel, and we were blessed. Sadly, when Taylor was one, Melissa, Mark, and Taylor moved to Arizona.

Melissa got a job with Johnson and Johnson and again was very successful. She made great money and received accolades for being in the top 10% of the sales reps for the company. We missed them terribly while they were in Arizona. We visited as often as possible, and Melissa flew back home with Taylor whenever she could. Even Melissa's grandma (my mother), who never flew, traveled with me to visit them. Grandma had a wonderful time, and I believe it was a highlight of her elder years! Yes, Melissa brought much joy to everyone's life!

While in Arizona, Melissa experienced some digestive problems and had her gallbladder removed. I went to be with her during surgery. She recovered from surgery, but her marriage deteriorated, and she got divorced. They moved back to Chicago, and we were able to help her with Taylor while she continued to work. While living as a single working mom, Melissa and her sister were injured in an automobile accident. The trauma from the accident caused pain and damage in her shoulder. She underwent shoulder surgery and thereafter was diagnosed with CRPS, Complex Regional Pain Syndrome. This disorder is characterized by chronic, severe pain. She required treatments and pain blocks for this painful disorder. Unfortunately, this created a kink in her highly successful work career.

The fact that she was unable to continue her fast-paced sales job did not put an end to her dreams of success, however. After all, she still had a beautiful daughter for which to provide. Melissa bought a small house for herself and Taylor. She also decided to get her master's degree in psychology to become a counselor. This was a job that she could perform that didn't require physical strength or travel. Her sister, Mary, moved in with her and helped her with Taylor. Life was becoming stable again. And then she met a man named Shawn.

Shawn was a single dad with one son, Max, living with him. He had experienced some hard times, as Melissa had. They had a connection. Melissa and Shawn were married in a lovely ceremony that included the children. The reception was enjoyed by all, and Melissa's life changed again. She gave birth to three more children in five years. One boy and two girls joined the family, making five children in total. Charlie was first born and has brought us much happiness. Sarah was next and is a sweet loving child. Katie, the baby, is a kind and caring child who gives the best hugs ever!

Life was good until Melissa went to doctor after giving birth to Katie. She was suffering from severe fatigue. She went to our beloved family doctor and was given a comprehensive physical to get to the bottom of the problem. At the same time my husband and I had bought a house in Florida to fulfill his lifelong dream of living in a warm climate. Our plan was to live as snowbirds until we retired. However, events happened that required us to change our plan. Ed, my husband, decided to move to Florida full time and build an insurance business. I was working full time at a local hospital and stayed in Illinois. Living apart was not ideal, but we talked everyday as well as travelled back and forth. During this time, Melissa was seeking medical help to uncover the cause of her ongoing tiredness. She did have five children and a husband whose career as an orthopedic surgeon required him to be gone often. This left her responsible for the children and the activities related to running the household. All of these responsibilities would make anyone tired!

Even as I worked full time, I was able to spend time with Melissa on the weekends and in the evenings. I treasured the time with her and our beautiful grandchildren. When I found a seemingly good job in Florida, we decided it was time for me to move full time with my husband. We planned to travel back to Illinois every 1–2 months to visit Melissa and the family. I secretly hoped they would buy a house down here for vacations so we would have more time together.

As the time approached for us to move, I gave my resignation, we made arrangements for a mover, and all was set. Then Melissa went for a muscle biopsy to finally get a diagnosis. I will never forget the day Melissa and Shawn picked me up from an appointment to give me a ride. They had just gotten the tentative results from the test, which indicated there were abnormal findings. She possibly had Pompe disease, and I felt like a knife stabbed me in the heart.

When they arrived, before I stepped into the car, Melissa whispered in my ear, "Don't talk about it. Shawn doesn't want to talk about it."

As I drove home that day I sobbed. My heart was broken as a million thoughts went through my head. *How could this happen to our daughter, Melissa Mae, who was "perfect"? Why would God do this to us? We are a loving, good family. Why us?* I wanted to hold Melissa in my arms as if she were a child again and cry together. When I talked to her the next day, I asked her if she wanted me to stay. She said that she wouldn't get involved with that decision.

Everything was so raw at this time; we really didn't know much about this rare disease. Ed and I did some research about the disease, treatment choices, etc. Melissa and Shawn decided to go with the enzyme replacement therapy, which meant she would receive the enzyme every other week. We trusted him to make the best decision for her since he is a doctor. Melissa started enzyme replacement therapy. She went through testing and started an exercise routine. Thankfully, her disease has not progressed as others, and I believe she is somewhat of a mystery to the Pompe doctors.

Melissa adheres to her five-hour enzyme infusion every other week at the hospital and has done well. She has always been a strong woman and is determined to be there for her children. She is an amazing mother, wife, daughter, sister, and friend. She now has started a group called Survivorship and is reaching out to all people who have survived something. Survivorship is a support group on Facebook that offers people the opportunity to discuss issues, ask questions, and get advice. She also interviews authors, business owners, and others on YouTube so they can share their knowledge about being a survivor.

We are blessed to have Melissa in our lives. Once again, I say she is perfect. Love you, Melissa.

- *9* -

My Journey with
Dr. Tim Lubenow

This is the start of our voyage together for a cure of Pompe disease, but it started with challenges, to say the least. This was the year of blessings and challenges for me and Dr. Tim Lubenow, who experienced the voyage from 2014–2016 with me. When I came about my diagnosis in 2013 and 2014, I sent the newspaper press releases to him so he could read about his former patient with a rare disease called Pompe disease. It is funny because my life was so different when I met Dr. Tim Lubenow in 2004. I thought that he was an amazing physician, but he had five children, which I said that I would *never* have. Now, I have five babies, and I'm married to a physician, who I said I would never marry. After Dr. Organic did not ask me to marry him, I was over physicians, but then I met Shawn, who wanted Taylor Mae and me. Never say never!

I have two very good friends who are pain physicians, but I owe my health Dr. Tim Lubenow. I drive an hour just to see him. He is the director of at one of the largest pain centers in the United States, Rush Medical Center.

When I sent him the newspapers, he was surprised, but he already knew that I had Pompe disease. I had sent him a letter, along with my diagnosis and the newspaper articles. After I sent the letter, I asked him if I could be his patient again, and he said of course. He knew a very little about Pompe disease, but he watched the movie *Extraordinary Measures* and asked me why I was not like the other patients in the movie. My medical case confused the physicians around the suburbs here in Barrington, but Dr. Tim Lubenow began to read and learn about Pompe disease on his own to help me. We even met with the Lumizyme sales representative to answer questions about my disease. This disease is so rare that few have heard of it, but Dr. Tim Lubenow learned everything he could by reading my test results, consulting with neuromuscular physicians, and asking the Genzyme sales representative. Now that is a perfect physician.

Dr. Tim Lubenow asked for my diagnosing information. I finally gave it to him in December 2015. It was not because I did not want to, but because all of my information was lost; yes, missing. It actually took years to find all of the information because one diagnosing test called a dry blood spot was lost at the Mayo Clinic, and it was never presentenced to the world's leading geneticists or to Dr. Tim Lubenow. This is definitely an example of being your own health advocate and keeping track of your test results, especially if you have one of the rarest diseases out there called Pompe disease. I was able to supply my champion with the results, and so we began fighting the fight together. The following is the story of how all that worked out.

January 2013

I started in his office with a major decision, which was neck surgery and what to do with my neck. Dr. Chow, who is my spinal orthopedic surgeon and annually checks on my scoliosis, said we needed to do a triple cervical fusion. I had an opinion from one of my husband's partners, who is fabulous, and he advised me to go to Dr. Chow because my neck was a complicated issue. I had many herniated disks and intense headaches. I saw Dr. Chow, and he agreed that my neck needed to be fixed, but it was going to encompass a lot of rehabilitation, and Pompe disease would have a major flare-up. There was also concern with my slightly abnormal pulmonary function tests (lung tests) during surgery. My breathing is slightly affected, and it can be an issue during surgery.

"Did you visit with one of the best pain physicians in the world, Dr. Tim Lubenow?"

"Yes, I know him, and we refer patients to him," I said. I do not know why I did not mention that he had treated me many years before.

Dr. Tim Lubenow was booked up for months, but he saw me the next day as a patient. The only thing that I knew to do was to have a talk with Dr. Tim Lubenow, who was concerned about me having a major surgery with Pompe disease, and I trusted his opinion after he treated me for Complex Regional Pain Syndrome so many years ago. He reviewed my imaging studies, which included CT Scans and MRIs, in his office with his team of students. He looked at me, and he said to me, "Melissa, this will be a major surgery, and you will not have the entire motion of your neck. Your pulmonary function tests are not normal, and yours are not because you have Pompe disease. I'm concerned about your outcome as your physician and your Pompe disease. Yes, your neck needs to be fixed, but how? Let me look at the imaging studies and see what I can advise you to do."

This appointment was for two hours. Dr. Tim Lubenow and his followers looked through my studies, and he said that we may have options with this surgery. "Let's look at all the places of pain besides your right arm," he said. This was a week before my mother-in-law and my mother were flying into Chicago for the neck procedure. Dr. Lubenow and I agreed that I would spend one night in the hospital and go home after. I'm stubborn, and I made the physicians release me two hours after the procedure. My loving husband wanted to care of me because he is a physician and surgeon, who I swore that I would never marry. I laughed, and I said that my mother is a RN and my husband is a surgeon, so they could handle me. I wanted to be home with my children.

The noise for a month was awful. At the postsurgical visits Dr. Lubenow asked me what my symptoms were and how I was doing.

"It's the same as Complex Regional Pain Syndrome," I answered.

"Okay, just hang in there because it will get better for you," he assured me. "I will watch your scoliosis yearly, and you can get the white board x-ray at Dr. Chow's office." He added, "You have muscle disease, and you may need a lumbar surgery, so I will check in with you in office visits every two weeks, and then we can do monthly visits. I can manage your pain with medication and monthly visits."

Dr. Tim Lubenow does not want me to be on medications, but I have muscle disease and spinal disease, so we do the best we can with my quality of life. We didn't have an option.

"How is your stomach doing?" he asked, which was embarrassing, but he is my doctor, and I have to be honest with him. Dr. Tim Lubenow was looking at the entire picture of Pompe disease when he could just be looking at the medications and imaging studies. He asked to see the diagnosing information about my Pompe disease, but I did not have it. I showed him the genetic tests, and I told him that I was going to Duke, which is Pompe central, to visit with Dr. Priya Kishani and my girlfriend Chrissie in April 2015. Lastly, I mentioned to him that Taylor was going away to the University of Iowa as one of the only females in the program. He said that his youngest son, Tommy, was in the program.

I told the doctor of my lumbar back pain, and we completed imaging studies. I had the choice to have a lumbar fusion. He mentioned a device that he frequently surgically implanted called a Medtronic spinal stimulator. It involved a study and psychological exam, and if the study was positive, than we would do a permanent one.

Cool, I thought, *no surgery, and I get an innovative device with Pompe disease instead of back surgery.* I had neck pain with the neck surgery and didn't want more pain. He implanted the spinal stimulator, which worked better than my neck surgery, but I still have a lot of pain from my neck and muscle tremors. There are some days that I cannot walk because it hurts so badly.

Dr. Palmer does not know how bad my neck still is, but Dr. Tim. Lubenow does, and he can refer back to the studies. He helped me a lot by implanting the stimulator and saying no to low back surgery. Now I do have a scar on my back, but God gave me great skin, and it healed up nicely.

During the next visit he said, "In 2015, let's look at your Pompe tests, Melissa."

"I do not have them. I asked the RN from Lurie Children's, and she only had part of my results," I explained.

After many phone and calls to Mayo Healthcare they were able to locate my lab results from when I was thirty-six years old. I brought Dr. Tim Lubenow the tests, and we reviewed them together. He asked me if any geneticists had seen my test together, and I simply stated no, they had not. After that, Dr. Tim Lubenow looked up the two largest facilities in the world and the best Pompe physicians. He asked me to confirm my enzyme levels. Let's solve this mystery.

"Your enzyme levels are really low, and you have rebounded over the past six years," he said. "It may benefit you to visit these two Pompe physicians."

Why?" I asked.

"Because I see you as strong, but your testing shows negative enzymes."

I agreed, and together we are redoing the initial diagnosing tests to get some answers about my Pompe disease. Dr. Tim Lubenow is responsible for gathering the initial Pompe testing recently and motivating me to get an opinion and an answer. Why am I strong? Why am I thriving? What is behind his patient's science and me? Dr. Tim Lubenow wanted to know why. As a trained anesthesiologist with a specialty pain management in my main symptoms, he needed answers. We found out from Duke Lenox Baker Children's Hospital that I'm a mystery to this disease. My enzyme levels are five percent. It is severe.

I received this e-mail regarding my enzyme levels in 2016. Do I have a genetic mutation kicking in or another enzyme? We do not know, and no one does.

Dr. Tim Lubenow pushes me, but he sees me thrive. After that, I started a foundation that required a lot of my time. I did not listen to my physicians of Pompe disease and started exercising again. He did not see me as my lab work portrayed me. I was excreting muscle and was deficient in GAA. He did see symptoms; he saw me as different from the other Pompe patients that he had read about and the muscular dystrophy patients that he works with. Dr. Tim Lubenow wanted to know why I was different from others. With his encouragement, we set out to challenge the initial diagnosis of Pompe disease, and we wanted to find out why I am different from the other patients in the medical literature with moderate Pompe disease.

Well we did receive an answer from Duke University upon the retesting of the skin fibroblast. Yes, my pain is real, and Mayo was correct six years ago. I have incredibly low enzymes, and I will spend a lifetime on Lumizyme, which means every other week in the hospital.

To: Melissa Mae Palmer
<melissataylor72@hotmail.com>
Subject: GAA enzyme results

Hi Melissa,

Your skin biopsy GAA enzyme results are
back. They were consistent with a diagnosis
of Late Onset Pompe. Any value at or under
40% activity (yours is 5.18%)is consistent
with LOPD. Infantile disease shows a GAA
value of under 1% to give you some
perspective of severity. This value along with
your genetic testing results, and clinical
presentation, this warrants treatment with
Lumizyme. As we discussed before, you can
consider a trial break from Lumizyme if you
feel that you are not benefitting on a clinical
level, however, your results are consistent
with the diagnosis and are enough to
warrant treatment. GAA activity in the skin is
the most reliable tissue, as results in blood
can be in the normal range while the skin
result is in the deficient range (as yours
was).

Please let me know if you have additional
questions.

<image001.png>

My liver enzymes are normal now. Why, we do not know. I do not have breathing problems with frequent lung infections, trouble with swallowing, inability to sleep and exercise, and all my friends with Pompe do and are on BiPAP or CPAP. I am not. I can walk unassisted, and they cannot. Travel has been a challenge because I enjoy it, but each time I do it, I end up with a virus. I went on a thirty-one-hour voyage last year with my beautiful family to see lions and tigers in South Africa. The physicians know that Dr. Tim Lubenow is my treating physician, and they all said that it is up to Lubenow. He told me, "It will be difficult, but you can do it one time." I was happy that I was able to share the experience with my children and my husband, but it was rough on me. The next voyage we are deciding on is Mexico, and I do not know if I can do it. Dr. Tim Lubenow and I are trying to decide on this. I do know this, however: I am a survivor, and my lifetime mystery was solved. We all are!

Tips for Survivorship Part 2 by Melissa Mae Palmer

1. Count your blessings because we can always make lemonade from lemons.
2. Prayer. I pray to my children every single night: now I lay me down to sleep, I pray the Lord. Believe in our savior. We pray for family each other and friends.
3. Survivorship is a process that we all endure.
4. Always keep your medical records in a file, like my Mayo dry blood spot test, which indicated no enzyme was lost.
5. Be your own health advocate and find a champion physician. Believe in yourself. You are worth it!
6. Males and females, do not let anyone say to you that it is in your head. What we feel is *real*.
7. Males and females, we are all survivors of something. Remember to *fight* in life because it will and can be positive when you are ill.

8. Find a satisfying purpose. I dedicate my time to charity, and I even had my own charity, which I donated to the hospital where I receive my hamster enzyme.

I have tried to build Pompe awareness in every way I can. The following are some of the things I have done to help find a cure for Pompe:

1. I have done media interviews on Margaret McSweeney's *Kitchen Chat* to raise funds for the Duke's 2016 conference. Through awareness of this rare genetic disease, we were able to bring donations to Duke.
2. I have raised money for the sick children at Duke.
3. My daughters Katie and Sarah put together twenty-five gift bags to the Dukes Infantile Conference in 2016.
4. I have donated iPads from the Palmer Family and the Lubenow family to children with Pompe disease in 2015.
5. I have donated assisted toilets to adults.
6. I donated funds to an adult basket cheer-up Pompe project in 2013.
7. I have donated funds to women and men who need medical supplies for basic daily living.

- *10* -

Melissa Mae Palmer: A Mystery Unsolved

Is Melissa Mae Palmer's Pompe Disease Solved?

There are some questions that I cannot get answers for.

1. What does it mean to have the only genetic code seen in mankind since a male in medical literature in the 1950s?
2. I was told by a leading genetic physician that I'm physically strong, but I make next to no enzymes: 5.18% Why?
3. During pregnancy I had zero disease symptoms? Why?
4. My liver enzymes are lower each year. Why?
5. My symptoms are fatigue and pain. They are not breathing, walking, and heart troubles. Why, with so little enzyme?
6. My parents and I were told by a leading genetic research physician that I could possibly have another enzyme protecting me or a genetic mutation. Which one is it?

7. Prednisone has made my symptoms better, and that is the only difference.
8. My hexose tetrasaccharide has improved over the past three years. Why?
9. My liver enzymes are almost normal. Why?

Will these questions with one of the rarest diseases of mankind be answered? We may never know.

- 11 -

From the Perspective of Dr. Tim Lubenow

My name is Dr. Tim Lubenow, and I am an international expert on Complex Regional Pain Syndrome. I spend a great deal of his time lecturing physicians and training them to understand CRPS for fully. I have served as an expert witness for thirty years for CRPS and other anesthesia matters; I have also trained medical residents and fellows for thirty years. I become interested in pain management because I saw it as an opportunity to help other overcome painful medical conditions. Because I want to not only help patients, but also doctors serving patients, I have authored twelve book chapters and written around twenty medical manuscripts to better circulate the knowledge I'm gaining in the field.

The following is a detailed report I have written about a very special patient, Melissa Mae Palmer. I wrote this in April 2016. It helps explain more accurately the kind of pain she has experienced for years as well as the ways I have been able to treat it.

Melissa Mae Palmer was a twenty-six-year-old woman, a professional sales representative for a pharmaceutical company, who was involved in a motor vehicle accident in May 2001. She was hit head-on in the motor vehicle accident, and her right shoulder came to hit the steering wheel. She went on to develop persistent right shoulder pain that did not heal with conservative care.

She was evaluated by an orthopedic surgeon who felt that she had impingement syndrome of the right shoulder. She underwent one initial arthroscopic shoulder surgery for treatment of the impingement syndrome, but this did not improve. Rather, she had the complication of having some laxity of the shoulder, which required a second surgery one month later to, in essence, tighten up the shoulder. She continued to have persistent pain, and then in March 2002, almost two years after the initial accident, she had a third surgery because she still had significant pain but could not lift her shoulder above 90°.

Following the March 2002 surgery, she began to develop additional symptoms of a neurological pain condition called complex regional pain syndrome (CRPS) or reflex sympathetic dystrophy (RSD). The symptoms that she began to have were a pallor, a sort of pale discoloration of the arm, loss of hair on her arm, increased sweating of the right upper extremity, and a significant hypersensitivity to simple tactile touch. She had muscle atrophy develop and had coolness of the right upper extremity. These are all the characteristic symptoms of CRPS.

The condition known as complex regional pain syndrome (CRPS) was first described during the American Civil War. Not coincidentally, as a result of advances in battlefield medicine during this time, soldiers were surviving from wounds that formerly would have claimed their lives. Yet many carried with them a constant reminder of the war: severe, crippling, neurologic pain that long outlasted the healing of their wounds. This condition was termed "causalgia." Veterans were not the only ones affected. It was noted at the turn of the century that patients could develop similar sequelae following trivial injuries, which might evolve into osteoporosis and atrophy at the site of injury. Rene Leriche was the first to implicate the sympathetic nervous system as a factor in the condition, and the term "reflex sympathetic dystrophy" (RSD) was introduced to reflect the proposed disruption in the sympathetic nervous system to the affected area. Over time, many different names have been applied to the features that culminate in the syndrome.

Prior to 1986, no formalized descriptive criteria existed for RSD. In 1986, the IASP proposed a formal classification of the condition. However, the description lacked rigorous diagnostic criteria, and many neuropathic pain conditions were erroneously given the diagnosis of RSD, specifically those resistant to traditional treatments. In 1994, the IASP published diagnostic criteria for CRPS that focused on clinical diagnosis from patient history, symptom description, physical signs, and pain. These diagnostic criteria were:

- The presence of an initiating noxious event or a cause of immobilization (Type I) or continuing pain or allodynia after a nerve injury, not necessarily limited to the distribution of the injured nerve (Type II).
- Continuing pain, allodynia, or hyperalgesia in which the pain is disproportionate to any known inciting event.
- Evidence at some time of edema; changes in skin blood flow or abnormal sudomotor activity in the region of pain.
- The diagnosis is excluded by the existence of other conditions that would otherwise account for the degree of pain and dysfunction.

This new taxonomy divided CRPS into type I and type II, distinguished by their inciting events. Type I (formerly RSD) follows a soft tissue injury, and CRPS II (causalgia) follows a well-defined nerve injury. The new term encompassed the many facets of the syndrome, including the complexity of the varied presentations; the distribution of symptoms; the presence of pain usually out of proportion to the inciting trauma; and the fact that it is a syndrome, which denotes the constellation of signs and symptoms. CRPS specifically addresses the varied contribution of the sympathetic nervous system.

Still, the revised IASP criteria suffered a lack of specificity, meaning that although they reliably identified many cases of CRPS, many non-CRPS cases were given the diagnosis incorrectly. This lack of specificity stemmed from the fact that the diagnostic IASP criteria for CRPS could be met entirely based on patient reporting of symptoms, allowing the clinician great leeway in interpreting whether the condition was out of proportion to injury.

Budapest Criteria

In direct response to these limitations, an international consensus panel was convened in Budapest in 2003 with the goal of recommending improvements to the IASP criteria. These modified criteria, henceforth known as the Budapest criteria, mandated that both historical and physical exam features in the following four key areas be present at the time of diagnosis.

1. At least one sign at time of evaluation in *two or more* of the following categories
   - *Sensory:* Reports of hyperesthesia and/or allodynia
   - *Vasomotor:* Reports of temperature asymmetry and/or skin color changes and/or skin color asymmetry
   - *Sudomotor/edema:* Reports of edema and/or sweating changes and/or sweating asymmetry
   - *Motor/trophic:* Reports of decreased range of motion and/or motor dysfunction (weakness, tremor, dystonia) and/or trophic changes (hair, nail, skin)
2. Continuing pain, disproportionate to any inciting event
3. At least one symptom in *three of the four* following categories
   - *Sensory:* Evidence of hyperalgesia (to pinprick) and/or allodynia (to light touch and/or deep somatic pressure and/or joint movement)

- *Vasomotor:* Evidence of temperature asymmetry and/or skin color changes and/or asymmetry
- *Sudomotor/edema:* Evidence of edema and/or sweating changes and/or sweating asymmetry
- *Motor/trophic:* Evidence of decreased range of motion and/or motor dysfunction (weakness, tremor, dystonia) and/or trophic changes (hair, nail, skin)
4. No other diagnosis that better explains the signs and symptoms

Although the criteria set forth had been based on criteria that was empirically derived and previously published, they had never all been brought together in a single, unified diagnostic schema. Research since its publication suggests that the Budapest criteria lead to greater diagnostic consistency between clinicians and fewer diagnoses of CRPS. Research also suggests that these criteria improve on the existing IASP criteria. Clinicians most favor the Budapest criteria today.

The incidence and prevalence of CRPS varies. A population-based study of CRPS calculated the overall incidence of CRPS to be 26.2 per 100,000 person years, with the incidence of CRPS I to be 5.46 per 100,000 person years at risk and a prevalence of 20.57 per 100,000. The incidence of CRPS II has been reported at 0.82 per 100,000 person years at risk and prevalence of 4.2 per 100,000 person years.

Pathophysiology

Some disagreement exists regarding the mechanisms underlying CRPS. Likely more than one mechanism can describe or explain the pathophysiologic features. What is clear is that CRPS has a slight female predominance and a predilection for the extremities following trauma, fractures, and orthopedic surgeries. One observation regarding pathophysiology has been the marked upregulation of alpha-1 adrenoreceptors, which appears in the injured extremity. These newly expressed alpha-1 receptors spread along skin, muscle, and nerve tissue. These then augment depolarization in nerve and muscle tissue, resulting in an amplification effect of any stimuli. This accounts for the increase in pain when a patient has an increase in either endogenous or exogenous catecholamines, such as during times of stress.

Other theories have been put forth implicating peripheral mechanisms as well as central mechanisms for CRPS. In CRPS II, biochemical, physiological, and morphological changes occur in the injured primary afferent neurons. The changes likely become permanent if the axotomized afferent neurons do not regenerate to their target tissue. This causes many dorsal root ganglion cells (DRG) with unmyelinated afferent fibers to die. The loss of DRG cells leads to degeneration of the centrally projecting afferent axons and to denervation of dorsal horn neurons. This induces secondary changes in the central representations (in the spinal cord, brain stem, thalamus, and forebrain).[1]

In contrast, although CRPS I presents with symptoms similar to those seen in CRPS II, it usually does not present with a preceding nerve injury. Jänig et al. hypothesized that in CRPS I, central representations of the sensory, autonomic, and somatomotor systems account for the clinical presentation. Later work, however, has unified the theories, arguing that CRPS, particularly type I, is a systemic disease of neuronal systems; the somatosensory system, the sympathetic nervous system, the somatomotor system, and peripheral (vascular, inflammatory) systems.

Clinical Features

CRPS is a painful and debilitating disorder primarily affecting one or more extremities. The key features in CRPS are spontaneous pain, allodynia, hyperalgesia, edema, temperature change, abnormal vasomotor and sudomotor activity, trophic changes, and motor dysfunction.

---

[1]   https://www.asra.com/pain-resource/article/6/complex-regional-pain-syndrome#r14

Although CRPS most frequently affects the limbs, it can occur anywhere in the body. A CRPS-like syndrome may be observed in patients with certain neoplasms (e.g., lung, breast, central nervous system, and ovarian cancers) and in patients after myocardial infarction or strokes.

Spontaneous Pain

Patients suffering from CRPS may describe burning, throbbing, squeezing, aching, or shooting pain localized deep in the tissue. This usually follows tissue injury to an extremity but is characteristically disproportionate in severity, duration, and extent of that expected from the clinical course of the initial injury.[2] Pain can be sympathetically mediated (relieved by sympathetic blockade), sympathetically independent (not relieved by sympathetic blockade), or mixed. CRPS varies in quality from a deep ache to a sharp stinging or burning sensation. Often patients report that environmental (cold, humidity) and emotional (anxiety, stress) factors worsen the pain. Cutaneous hypersensitivity presents as pain on contact with clothing or exposure to a cool breeze. The involved extremity is often guarded, even from the examining physician, and neglect of hygiene is common in the affected limb.

Evoked Pain

Patients frequently experience pain from innocuous tactile stimuli (allodynia) and have an increased response to painful stimuli (hyperalgesia). All patients suffer from hyperalgesia, predominantly to mechanical stimuli or on joint movement. One third (higher incidence in chronic stages) suffer from severe allodynia (brush-evoked pain), a hallmark of central nociceptive sensitization.

---

2   https://www.asra.com/pain-resource/article/6/complex-regional-pain-syndrome-r18

Sudomotor Changes and Edema

Although sometimes absent at presentation, marked edema can develop in the affected limb and be severe enough to lead to functional loss of the limb. Edema in the painful region gives a glossy and smooth appearance to the skin (see figure 1). Notable limb edema has been reported in 80% of CRPS patients. Sudomotor abnormalities range from hyperhidrosis to bone-dry skin and have been reported in 53% of patients.

As mentioned before, the diagnostic criteria set forth by IASP had a high sensitivity (0.98) but low specificity (0.36).[3] A low-specificity diagnostic tool leads to a high level of false positives and misdiagnoses. Many conditions mimic CRPS, and the lack of high diagnostic specificity may lead to inclusion, improper treatment, or delay in appropriate treatment.

The following should be used for differential diagnosis of CRPS:

- Fracture, sprain, strain
- Traumatic vasospasm
- Cellulitis
- Lymphedema
- Raynaud's disease
- Thromboangiitis obliterans
- Erythromelalgia
- Deep vein thrombosis

The Budapest modifications to the IASP original criteria allow a diagnosis of CRPS to be accurate in up to 88% of cases and a diagnosis of non-CRPS neuropathic pain likely to be accurate in 97% of cases. Additionally, the Budapest criteria retain the sensitivity of the IASP criteria (0.99) but with markedly higher specificity (0.68). Recent work has provided external validation of the Budapest criteria as being superior to the IASP criteria and

---

[3] https://www.asra.com/pain-resource/article/6/complex-regional-pain-syndrome–r37

suggest that it is likely the most rigorous diagnostic tool we have in identifying cases of CRPS.

A general definition of the syndromes of CRPS describes an array of painful conditions that are characterized by a continuing (spontaneous or evoked) regional pain that is seemingly disproportionate in time or degree to the usual course of any known trauma or other lesion. The pain is regional (not in a specific nerve territory or dermatome) and usually has a distal predominance of abnormal sensory, motor, sudomotor, vasomotor, or trophic findings. The syndrome shows variable progression over time.

Debate exists regarding the best way to assess the various signs and symptoms necessary to make the diagnosis of CRPS. CRPS lacks a single objective test for its diagnosis, but a number of diagnostic tests may assist in determining the likelihood of the syndrome.

Treatment

Pharmacological Therapy

The foundation of proper CRPS treatment lies in functional restoration, pain control, and psychotherapy. Therapeutic goals focus on optimizing the functional state of the extremity through physical therapy and psychotherapy and on reducing stimulus-evoked pain and pain associated with extremity movement. The initiation of early functional restorative therapy is critical and correlates with improved outcomes. An algorithm has been proposed (see figure 5) outlining treatment modalities, and therapy is directed at managing the signs and symptom of the disease.

Antidepressants

Both tricyclic and dual-inhibitor antidepressants have demonstrated efficacy in treating a variety of neuropathic pain conditions. The effect of tricyclic antidepressants is multimodal. They antagonize calcium channels, sodium channels, and

N-Methyl-D-Aspartate (NMDA) receptors on spinal cord dorsal horn neurons. Additionally, at this site, they inhibit reuptake of serotonin and norepinephrine, and this constellation of effects likely underlies their benefit. Serotonin-norepinephrine reuptake inhibitors (SNRIs) inhibit the reuptake of both serotonin and norepinephrine and are often referred to as dual inhibitors. The literature does not yet support their use in CRPS, though their success in treating postherpetic neuralgia and diabetic peripheral neuropathy leads many to believe that these agents may reduce CRPS-associated pain. Although data is absent in the treatment of CRPS, the properties of the antidepressants may provide some symptom relief for the secondary consequences of the disease (e.g., an overweight, lethargic patient may benefit from an agent with more noradrenergic selectivity [desipramine], which may lead to appetite suppression). The sedating properties of amitriptyline also may be quite beneficial in patients with insomnia.

Anticonvulsants (Antiepileptics)

Antiepileptics for the treatment of CRPS have shown mixed results. Gabapentin (GBP) and pregabalin (PGB) are the most prescribed anticonvulsant drugs in the treatment of CRPS. GBP modulates the voltage-gated $\alpha2\delta$ subunit of the calcium channels, but its true analgesic mechanism of action remains unknown.

Mellick and Mellick presented a case series of six patients in which GBP provided satisfactory pain relief; a reduction of hyperpathia, allodynia, and hyperalgesia; reversal of skin and soft tissue manifestations; and improved sleep quality and sleep consolidation with far fewer nocturnal awakenings. In a prospective study, GBP was evaluated in twenty-two patients diagnosed with early stage CRPS. The outcome measures were spontaneous visual analog scale (VAS), provoked VAS, range of motion, and edema. Statistically significant improvements in spontaneous and provoked VAS were found but not in the other measures. In contrast, van de Vusse reported "mild effect on pain" with the use of GBP in patients with CRPS I.

Opioids

No long-term studies have been performed on oral opioids in the treatment of CRPS. Opioids should be considered in CRPS if pain limits the patient's participation in physical restorative therapies designed to establish, maintain, or enhance function of the affected extremity. Although opioids may be less effective for chronic neuropathic pain conditions than for nociceptive pain, the data for opioid use do support improvements in the quality of life for patients with neuropathic pain.

Recently, Agarwal studied the effect of transdermal fentanyl on pain and function in three groups of patients suffering from neuropathic pain (e.g., small fiber or diabetic peripheral neuropathy), CRPS, and postamputation pain in a prospective, open-label trial. Primary outcome measures included a change in pain intensity and daily activity, and secondary outcomes included pain relief, cognition, physical function, and mood. All three groups reported significant decreases in pain at study conclusion. The CRPS group reported a reduction of 2.4 ± 0.40 ($p < 0.001$) from baseline on a 0–10 numerical rating scale. Moreover, the CRPS group experienced a 37.5% increase in daily activities compared to baseline.

Calcium-Regulating Medications (Bisphosphonates and Calcitonin)

Bisphosphonates and pyrophosphate analogues recently have been promoted as effective agents for the treatment of CRPS, but the mechanism of action is unknown. These compounds (alendronate, pamidronate, clodronate) may inhibit bone resorption, and their effectiveness have been confirmed in randomized controlled trials.[4] Calcitonin, a hormone secreted by the parafollicular cells of the thyroid gland, acts on bone and kidneys to inhibit osteoclastic bone resorption and thereby reduces serum calcium and phosphate. Gobelet examined the efficacy of intranasal calcitonin

---

[4] https://www.asra.com/pain-resource/article/6/complex-regional-pain-syndrome–r51

in sixty-three patients with CRPS in a double-blind randomized study. Significant reduction in both pain at rest and in motion and increased mobility were reported. In a meta-analysis of pharmacologic treatments, Perez concluded that calcitonin could provide effective pain relief in CRPS patients.

Free Radical Scavenger

Dimethylsulfoxide (DSMO) and N-acetylcysteine (NAC) also have been shown to be effective in treating CRPS. The effectiveness and potency is variable, and their mechanism of action is unknown but may be related to their antioxidant properties.

Ketamine

The NMDA receptor antagonist ketamine has been used in the treatment of CRPS, although its use is controversial. Currently, two dosing schema are used. The first is a low-dose "awake" regimen consisting of IV ketamine 25–100 mg per hour administered daily either as an inpatient or outpatient and repeated over several days (e.g., 5–10 days). A recent placebo-controlled study by Schwartzman et al. (2009) administered ketamine to CRPS patients. The dose was 100 mg over four hours as an outpatient, repeated daily over ten days. Outcome measures included thermal sensitivity, dynamic and static allodynia, finger motor function, and deep-pressure pain thresholds. Patients were followed up at twelve weeks, and the ketamine group demonstrated statistically significant improvement in all primary outcome measures versus placebo. Patients required coadministration of clonidine and midazolam to attenuate unwanted side effects from ketamine (e.g., hallucinations).

A second dosing regimen involves periodically administering high-dose ketamine, 200–300 mg per hour, in a monitored anesthetic setting. Practitioners in Germany have medically induced comas in CRPS patients to administer extremely high doses of ketamine (3–5 mg/kg per hour) over five days, subsequently managing the emergence delirium on an outpatient basis. Such treatment is rarely reimbursed or approved by insurance companies in the United States.

Interventional Procedures

Sympathetic Nerve Blockade

Sympathetic blockade utilizing local anesthetics is performed for *treatment* of CRPS, not, as commonly believed, for diagnosis. Although poorly understood, the role of sympathetic nervous system dysfunction was previously presumed to be an essential component of the syndrome, but there is growing debate regarding the degree to which the sympathetic nervous system contributes to the clinical syndrome. A subset of CRPS patients may display sympathetically mediated pain and are more likely to receive pain relief from sympathetic blockade.

In a double-blind crossover study, Price investigated the effectiveness of local anesthetics in CRPS patients. An immediate effect on pain and mechanical allodynia was found, but the response was similar in the control group (saline). In a Cochrane Review, Cepeda revealed the scarcity of published data to support the use of local anesthetic sympathetic blockade as the gold standard for CRPS treatment. More recently, Yucel evaluated the effectiveness of stellate ganglion blockade in CRPS. The sympathetic blockade significantly improved VAS values and range of motion (ROM). Nerve blocks are recommended primarily to reduce pain and facilitate physiotherapy and functional rehabilitation. Those who obtain pain relief and improved ROM should continue with an extended series of repeat blocks.

Epidural Infusion

Continuous epidural infusion, often with local anesthetic and opioid (e.g., bupivacaine and fentanyl), is an effective analgesic option in the treatment of CRPS. The epidural catheter is placed sterilely under fluoroscopic guidance and aims to position the catheter tip on the affected side at the appropriate spinal segmental level. The catheter is tunneled under the skin for a distance of 3–5 inches and left in place for five days to twelve weeks. During infusion, the patient undergoes physiotherapy directed at restoration of function. Rauck et al. previously described in a randomized controlled fashion the efficacy of continuous epidural clonidine infusions for the treatment of refractory RSDD (CRPS) patients.

Neuromodulation

Studies show that conventional pain medications, physical therapy, and sympathetic blockade all have less-than-favorable results for CRPS treatment. Only one in five CRPS patients is capable of returning to a normal level of functioning. Spinal cord stimulation (SCS) is an intervention modality that may be used in patients with refractory pain. The proposed mechanism of SCS began with the gate theory advanced by Melzack and Wall in 1965. Specifically, the "gate" represents the termination of painful peripheral stimuli carried by C fibers (e.g., burning sensation) and thinly myelinated Aδ fibers (e.g., sharp, intense, tingling sensation) in the dorsal horn of the spinal cord. Large myelinated Aβ fibers (e.g., light touch, pressure, vibration, hair movement) also terminate in the dorsal horn. Melzack and Wall hypothesized that sensory input could be manipulated to close the "gate" to the transmission of painful stimuli. The mechanisms by which dorsal column stimulation modulate pain perception have yet to be elucidated; however, current understanding attributes pain reduction to the activation of large diameter afferent fibers (e.g., Aβ fibers) by electrical stimulation.

Symptoms of CRPS have been ranked the second-most frequent indicator for SCS therapy in the United States (postlaminectomy pain syndrome being the first indication). Pain relief as high as 70% has been reported with neurostimulation (e.g., SCS or peripheral nerve stimulation) when patients are properly selected. Spinal cord stimulation should be considered in the treatment algorithm when conservative therapies fail.

The literature supports the use of SCS in CRPS. For example, Kemler studied the effectiveness of spinal cord stimulation and physical therapy versus physical therapy alone in CRPS-affected patients. At six months, the SCS + physiotherapy group reported a significantly greater reduction in pain compared to the physiotherapy alone group. At twenty-four months, spinal cord stimulation resulted in improvement of long-term pain and health-related quality of life. At five years, despite the diminishing effectiveness of SCS over time, 95% of patients with an implant would repeat the treatment for the same result. Harke evaluated the long-term effect of SCS on functional improvement. When SCS was combined with concurrent physiotherapy, a reduction in deep pain and allodynia along with improvement in functional status and quality of life were found.

Intrathecal Drug Delivery

Data citing the benefits of intrathecal drug delivery systems (IDDS) are limited, although case reports and series indicate benefit in CRPS patients. An implantable pump is a viable consideration for patients who do not respond to SCS or have multiple sites of pain. Intrathecal medications have long been established as effective agents for treating refractory cancer pain since 1979. In a randomized control trial of two hundred patients with advanced cancer and refractory pain, Smith demonstrated the effectiveness of intrathecal opioid in a group of patients receiving both IDDS and medical management compared to medical management alone. The same has not been borne out in the treatment of CRPS. Alternatively, ziconitide (PRIALT®, Elan Pharmaceuticals Inc., San Diego, CA), a nonopioid analgesic, has shown some promise in the treatment of severe chronic nonmalignant pain, including CRPS.

Temperature Change

The acute clinical presentation of CRPS is rubor, increased skin temperature, and edema. In the more chronic stages of CRPS, skin color becomes cyanotic, and skin temperature decreases. Patients may describe the limb as mottled with dark, bluish, or pale-white discoloration (see figure 1). These temperature changes are secondary to autonomic disturbance, which ranges from sympathetic hypofunction (hot, red, and dry) to sympathetic hyperfunction (cold, blue, pale or mottled, and sweaty). A difference in skin temperature (either higher or lower by 1°C) is found in 42% of patients with CRPS, and a difference of more than 2.2°C has a sensitivity of 76% and a specificity of 93% for CRPS.[5]

Motor Disturbances

Movement disturbance in the affected limb may present as tremulousness, weakness, decreased range of movement, muscle spasms, and dystonia. Dystonia in the upper extremity is typified by fingers in fixed flexion. Dystonia in the lower extremity often presents as an equinovarus position of the foot (see figure 1). Hand or foot dystonia develops in about 10% of patients. Range of movement may be compromised on the affected side, and contractures may develop in severe cases. Patients also may report decreased range of motion (80%) or motor weakness in the affected limb (75%). Tremors have been reported in approximately 50% of patients. Approximately 20% of patients display cyclonic action in the affected area.

---

[5]   https://www.asra.com/pain-resource/article/6/complex-regional-pain-syndrome–r24

Trophic Changes

In latter stages of CRPS, fear for pain with movement can lead to disuse changes of the affected extremity, including osteoporosis visible by bone imaging. Patients may present trophic changes such as altered skin (hyperkeratosis), nail, or hair growth patterns (24%, 21%, and 18% of the patients, respectively). (See figures 2 and 3.) Changes to skin are likely to be more common than nail or hair changes.

Clinical Stages

Classically, CRPS was subdivided into three distinct, sequential, progressive stages, although recent work disputes this traditional staging and theorizes that patients are experiencing subtypes or subgroups. The classic stages are stage I (the acute early, warm stage), marked by pain/sensory abnormalities (e.g., hyperalgesia, allodynia), vasomotor dysfunction, edema, and sudomotor disturbance. Stage II (dystrophic stage) is proposed to occur three to six months after onset and is characterized by intensified pain and sensory dysfunction, continued vasomotor disturbance, and development of motor and trophic changes. Stage III (atrophic stage) is characterized by a relatively cold extremity with decreased pain and sensory disturbance, continued vasomotor disturbance, and markedly increased motor and trophic changes.

This staging categorization carries much less significance today as CRPS is typically recognized earlier than in the past. Many patients do not progress beyond stage I, or the timeframe in which they do advance is much more protracted than initially suggested. A multicenter cluster analysis was used to identify homogenous subgroups of patients with CRPS based on signs and symptoms and the duration of the disease. The derived subgroups were statistically distinct and suggested three possible CRPS subtypes: (1) a relatively limited syndrome with vasomotor signs predominating; (2) a relatively limited syndrome with predominately neuropathic pain and sensory abnormalities; and (3) a florid CRPS syndrome similar to "classic RSD" descriptions. The resulting CRPS subgroups did not differ significantly regarding pain duration, as might be expected in a sequential staging model. The IASP and Budapest diagnostic criteria acknowledge subgroups but do not make mention of the stages.

Pattern and Spread

CRPS does not affect a specific dermatome, and the spread of CRPS is quite common. Three patterns of spread have been characterized in the literature based on retrospective analysis (figure 4). Contiguous spread (CS) is the most common and is characterized by a gradual and significant enlargement of the area affected initially. Independent spread (IS) is characterized by the appearance of CRPS in a location that was distant and noncontiguous with the initial site (e.g., CRPS appearing first in a foot, then in the hand). Mirror-image spread (MS) is the appearance of symptoms on the opposite side in an area that is closely matched in size and location to the site of initial presentation. Schwartzman et al. reported CS in 31.1% of patients, MS in 11.5% of patients, ipsilateral extremity spread in 10.8% of patients, and contralateral extremity spread in 11.3% of patients.

Prognosis

CRPS can be marked by significant pain and chronicity. Controversy in the literature exists, with reports of spontaneous resolution of CRPS in some patients while many report continued symptoms. A recent report indicates that an average of 5.8 years after the initiating injury, CRPS patients continue to have significantly higher symptom and sign prevalence rates when compared to reference patients with the same precipitating injury. Most of the signs and symptoms became well-established after one year and might progress moderately with time.

Prognostic factors for a good or poor outcome of CRPS are not known, although coldness of the affected limb has been associated with longer disease duration and worse functional outcome. As with spontaneous resolution of symptoms, recurrence of symptoms may occur. It is a common belief that further trauma (e.g., surgery) to a previously affected extremity can reactivate CRPS, although this is not supported by literature data. The incidence of CRPS recurrence is estimated to be 10% or 1.8% per year at risk. A five-year follow-up study in patients with CRPS involving the upper extremity indicated that 26% of patients had to change their jobs, and nearly 30% of patients had to stop work for more than a year. However, 72% continued to work full time.

Summary

CRPS is a painful and debilitating disorder primarily affecting one or more extremities. A specific etiology has not been identified, and the poor understanding of the underlying pathophysiological abnormalities contribute to the difficulties in diagnosis and treatment. No single diagnostic test or single or combination of therapies are universally effective for CRPS. Currently, effective treatment of chronic neuropathic pain continues to be a clinical challenge because of the variability in presentation. Treatment of CRPS focuses on an early, aggressive, and multimodal approach that targets pain reduction and functional restoration. Presently, many of the medications used in the treatment of CRPS are approved for the treatment of other pain conditions. Continued research may reveal additional mechanisms of the disease leading to preventive measures and additional targets for drug activity.

Ms. Palmer began to search out alternative pain treatment providers because she was not improving with the orthopedic care that she was getting and the physical therapy. Her father found a doctor in Florida who specialized in the care and treatment of CRPS, and together they traveled there. This particular neurologist had treated her with injectable medications and gave her several injections, but because of the difficulty with transportation to and from Chicago and Florida, she then began to search out alternative pain treatment providers in the Chicago area, and her orthopedic surgeon then referred her to my office for further care and management in 2002.

After my initial evaluation, I felt that she had CRPS of the right upper extremity, and I recommended a series of injections to help her. The first series of injections were called stellate ganglion blocks. She had some partial response to these, which were coupled with physical therapy. Following that, she had some partial improvement but then went on to undergo another series of brachial plexus nerve blocks coupled with ongoing physical therapy in an effort to improve her symptoms. She had some further improvement but still had significant impairment and persistent, daily pain.

She was somewhat better and felt that she could continue on with her training and education. She was in graduate school at the time, and in April 2004 she wanted to continue with graduate school and continued on with conservative care. At that time, she was a single mom with a five-year-old daughter.

She continued to improve with ongoing physical therapy and oral medications, and by February 2004 she was substantially improved to be able to get on with her life.

EPILOGUE

Other Voices of People I Love

Inspiration of a son's love and a poem with words that I read of admiration of my husband. My son Charlie (9) inspires me. This is about my ROCK of a husband!

—Melissa Mae Palmer

A Poem by Charlie

Someday, I will become an orthopedic surgeon like my dad.
And fix people's hips and knees and shoulders and feet and backs.
I will make the best out of my job.
And I might even fix famous people.
(My dad has fixed a famous athlete).
Right now, I am going into fiftth grade
and writing a someday poem
about my wishes and dreams
and everything I want to be and do.
(Like an orthopedic surgeon).

Someday, I will skydive out
of the biggest airplane ever
and feel the breeze blowing against my hair and fly.
I will flap my arms around like a bird
and do front flips and backflips in the air
then I will press the button on my suit
and a giant parachute will pop out
and I will gracefully glide to safety.
In the meantime, I ride my scooter
and feel the light breeze against my hair
as I wait and wait and wait
for my dad or mom to allow me to go skydiving or some other
awesome activity.

Someday, I will bungee jump off of a giant bridge
and then shoot to the moon
and then to it over and over again
until I'm so dizzy that even my eyes are wobbling.
And people will ask to interview me
for the first bungee jumping
moon shooter ever
and I will say, "No thanks
I did it for the fun, not the fame."
As for today, I slide down the stairs
on a gymnastics mat waiting and waiting
And waiting and waiting for my parents
to let me skydive or bungee jump.

Someday, I will be on my favorite game show
"Are You Smarter Than a Fifth Grader"
and I will win the one-million-dollar prize
and buy a ginormous mansion and
then use the rest on a pool and arcade.
Today, I answer trivia questions
on my iPad, get some right
and some wrong and practice
and practice.

ACKNOWLEDGMENTS

by Melissa Mae Palmer
and Dr. Tim Lubenow

I would like to take time to acknowledge the following people who have helped me become a survivor as I have battled a mystery illness that, even now that it is solved, remains mysterious. These people have encouraged me to write about what I want to write about and to tell my story to help others. I'm truly blessed for the support system that I have, and it always starts with the family and God. They also have given me the encouragement to write this book.

Edward and Nancy D'Agostin, who reside in Cape Coral, Florida, but are Illinois natives. They gave me the best childhood filled with love, and they have taught me the concept of togetherness, motherhood, and prayer. They did not know that they are recessive carriers of Pompe disease, nor that it mattered to me and would make my life different one single bit. I had the best childhood because I knew that I was emotionally supported and securely loved by them. My basic needs were always met by my parents. I still would have married Shawn, and we would have had children. Do my parents feel guilt about being genetic carriers of Pompe disease? Yes, but they *should not ever* because I have lived a life with supreme joy. With their love and nurturing, I had the confidence to live ill and succeed. I have my own priceless legacy: Team Palmer.

My children do not have this disease, but each of them are carriers, so the future of genetic testing will be important in their lives. When I was writing this book, my computer broke, and my father was the first person to run to Best Buy and purchase me a brand new laptop. I can't express my gratitude for their love and support. Those grandmothers in heaven are looking at me, and I know that they are giving me enzymes. We do know if my brother and sister have Pompe disease. Thank you to Billy and Mary for their sibling love while being the best auntie and uncle ever.

My legacy, which includes my five children—Taylor Mae, Max, Charlie, Sarah, Katie—and my husband, Dr. Shawn W. Palmer. **Team Palmer** inspires me! Shawn is with me and loving me every day and night. I admire him, and I still enjoy his deep-green eyes that stare at me.

Lynda Yost, the most amazing and dynamic woman that I have ever met. You are so dynamic, and I look up to you always and guidance through writing this book. You have showed me how females can be it all. I love the feminine role in life, and you have it with your career and family. You gave me your priceless time, and I will forever appreciate you. I want to be just like you!

Judy and Katharine Grubbe. Judy is a female business owner in Barrington Hills, Illinois, who took this manuscript and organized it. She said that it was a beautiful story and to finish it. She is a mother of one of Taylor's friends from high school.

The Kappa Kappa Gamma sisters, who have been there for Taylor at college. The sisters have supported Taylor and are such good females to society.

Dr. Tim Lubenow, thank you for encouraging me through this voyage of writing and for giving me your time and interest in Pompe disease while encouraging me not to progress with illness. You can help a person achieve their goals in life. You are one in a billion! You were correct; there is no reason for me to sit in the wheelchair or rocking chair like my grandma and not to share this story! Dr. Tim Lubenow wants me to walk and live until I'm seventy. He is my champion in this lifetime. Thank you, Rush University.

Dr. Richard McDonough, thank you for a lifetime of care and never saying that the illness was in my head. Also, you diagnosed my Pompe disease, and you have championed me.

Debbie Overton from Good Shepherd Hospital, you have taken care of me and have been my friend for over two decades; you know my deepest secrets. I love you!

Margaret McSweeney of KitchenChat, thank you for your charitable interview on Pompe disease and bringing awareness to this with you syndicated beautiful channel (www.kitchenchat.info margaret mcsweeny@mcsweeny Twitter).

Thank you Mark Mingle for being so knowledgeable in this industry and an asset to my first book.

The friends, families, and businesses of Barrington, Illinois, and the zip code 60010. We live in the best pay-it-forward community on earth. All of the parents and families ask, "How are you feeling?" and are really great to Team Palmer.

Chrissie Mena, for her writing in this book as a friend.

Laura Billor. I would like to thank the best friend in my entire life, Laura Billor. I met her when Taylor was in first grade. The girls grew up together and we became so close. She is my assistant and Godmother to my younger children. Secret to survivorship is having your best friend, her husband and two children support you. We have been best friends for 14 years. I love her to pieces. She acts like a second mother to Katie. Everyone needs a Godmother like Laura.

Eleanor Anne Sweet. Thank you, Eleanor Anne Sweet, for helping me with my book.

I would like to thank Barrington Children's Charities in Barrington IL. For impacting the lives of children positively.

To the American Cancer Society – Relay For Life, Barrington Il. You do so much for people with cancer. You are the best charity and you make a difference.

Barrington Junior Womens Club, you all are fantastic ladies that helped other so much by dedicating your time for charitable causes.

I would like to thank Bataille Academie of the Danse and Ms. Dee Dee. I would like to thank Ms. Dee Dee for making everyone's mother's day special.

Special thanks to the Daily Herald and writer Douglas T. Graham for bringing awareness in Pompe Disease and Melissa Mae Palmer.

Special thanks to my suburban life and writer Stephanie Kohl.

I would like to thank Chicago Tribune and Melissa Mae Palmer for bringing awareness to Melissa Mae Palmer.

I would like to thank my brother and sister. Mary is a special soul that I adore and Billy is the uncle that everybody dreams about. Nicole, her daughter is like my child and Mickey as well.

Thanks to the Kea's, the Grimes and the D'Agostin's

I would like to thank a special person, Dr. Zina from the Community Church of Barrington for her special prayer which we all need.

I would like to thank my special friend who took the photos, Thomas Balsamo of Barrington Il. Portraits by Thomas. He is dear to me in many ways.

I have a girlfriend named Cory Flahaven and her husband Jason and Kendal, they are very special to me and dear to my heart.

Thank you, Dad, owner of Freedom Capital Freedom, Freedom Premier Financial Group, Cape Coral, Florida. You inspire me to work hard in spite of all these illnesses. I promise you that I will keep trying.

I'd like to express my sincere thanks to my lovely wife, Tish, and five great children, Chris, Jen Madeline, Cassie, and Tommy. Without their love and support I would not have been able to achieve many of the career goals I have sought. I would like to thank Melissa Mae Palmer for being an inspiration to so many people. Practicing pain medicine has many challenges and is not always rewarding, but when one special person with not just one chronic medical condition-causing pain—but several—can still exemplify an encouraging, inspiring attitude about life, work then becomes an gratifying fulfilling activity that doesn't seem like work.

To connect with Melissa Mae Palmer, please join her website at www. melissapalmersurvivorship.com and Facebook site Survivorship

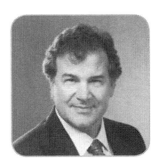

If you have any questions,
regarding Melissa Mae Palmer medial case
please contact Dr. Tim Lubenow on complex
regional pain syndrome, and her unique case
of Pompe Disease. We would like to find
the first cure for muscular dystrophy.

Please email me at
findapompecure@gmail.com
or www.mysecretsofsurvivorship.com
or facebook Survivorship.

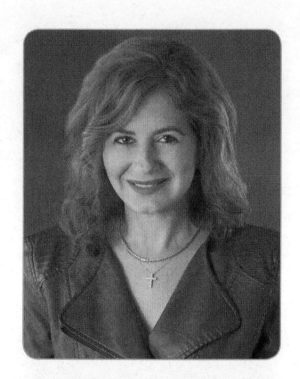

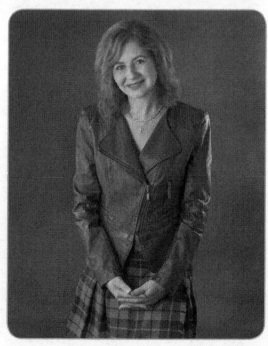

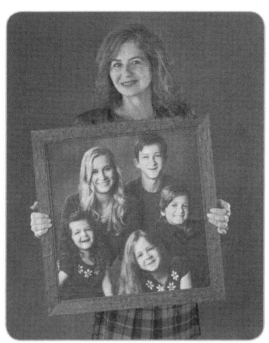

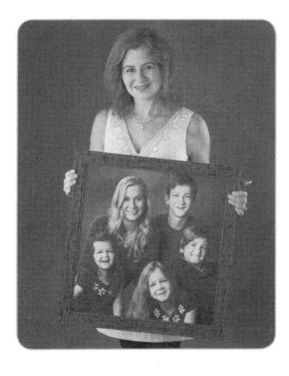

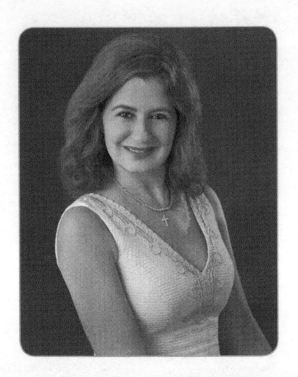

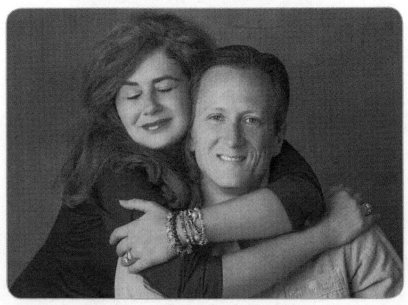

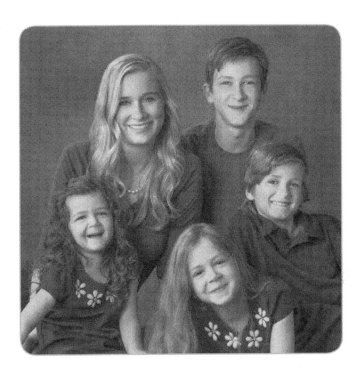

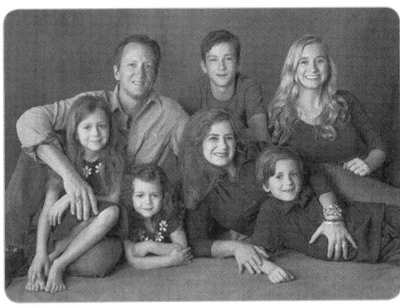

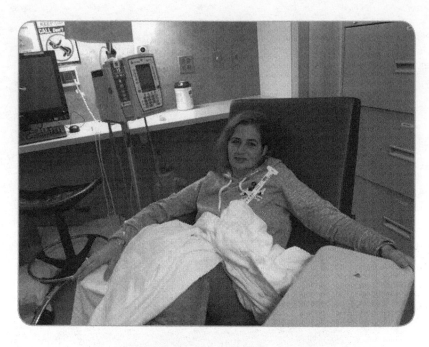

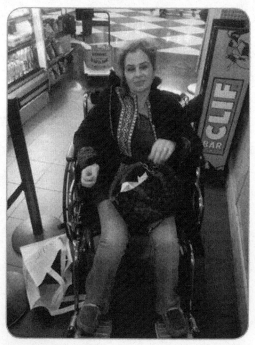

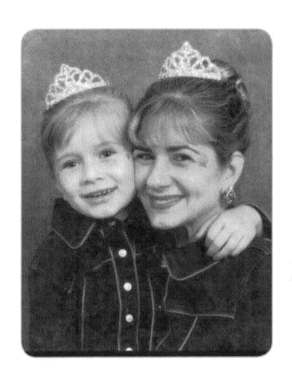

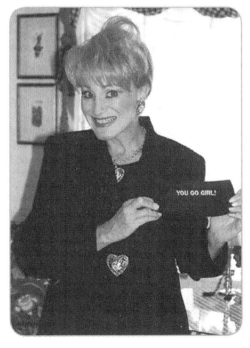

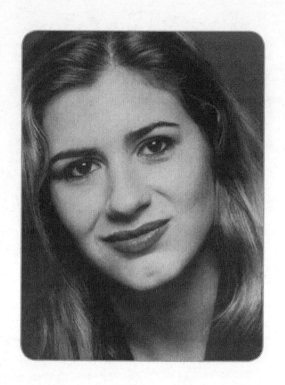

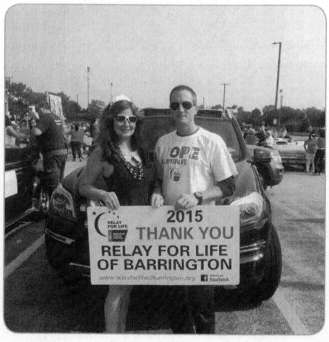

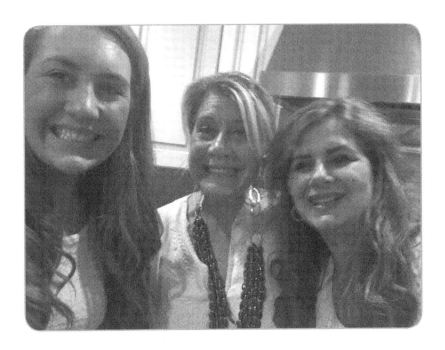

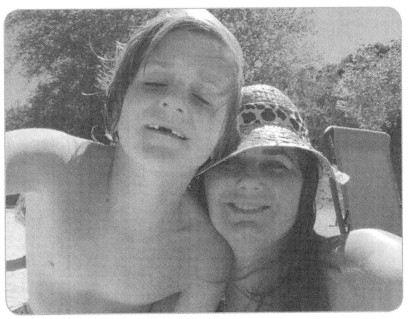

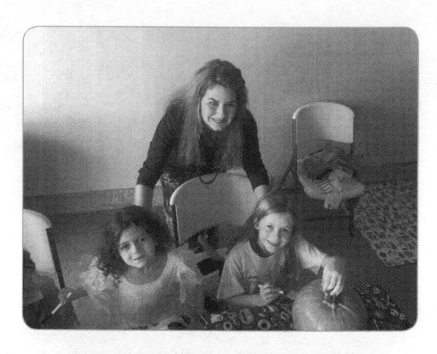

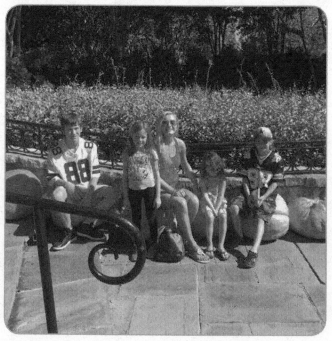

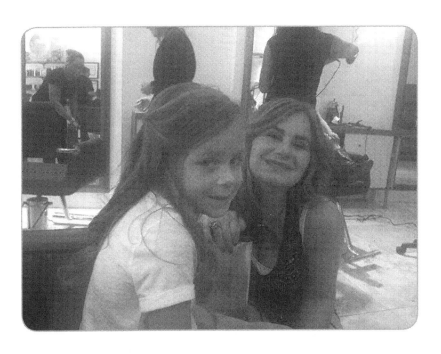

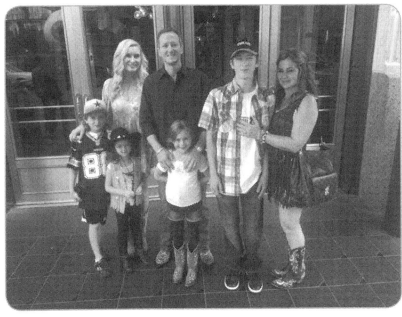

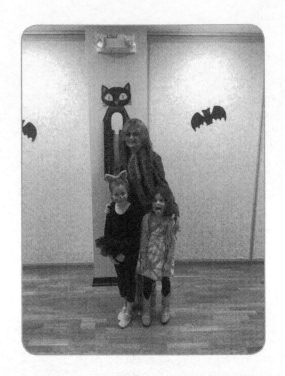

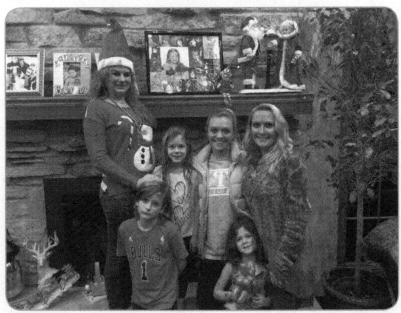

64067226R00084

Made in the USA
Lexington, KY
27 May 2017